TOTAL WOMAN'S FITNESS GUIDE

TOTAL WOMAN'S FITNESS GUIDE

By Gail Shierman, Ph.D. &
Christine Haycock, M.D.

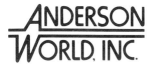

ANDERSON
WORLD, INC.

Library of Congress Cataloging in Publication Data

Shierman, Gail.
  Total woman's fitness guide.

  1. Physical fitness for women. 2. Exercises for
women. 3. Women—Health and hygiene. I. Haycock,
Christine, joint author. II. Title.
RA781.S55   613.7'045   78-23355
ISBN 0-89037-163-6

Second Printing, December 1981

Anderson World, Inc.
Mountain View, CA

This book is dedicated to all women who care about themselves.

Contents

Acknowledgments

The authors acknowledge the following women who helped complete this book: Mandy Woodford, Maureen Murphy, Maranda Maier, Pauline Stockdale, and Diane Staggs.

1

Fitness For Every Woman

Although many books have been written about fitness and about running as a sole means of achieving fitness, few have been written just for women and fewer have concerned themselves with women's alternatives for achieving fitness. For the many women who do not like to run or cannot run for one reason or another, there are many other ways of achieving fitness. In the same regard, the abundance of much incorrect information given women about diet, exercise, and weight control has led many women to invest a great deal of time, energy, and money into an exercise or activity program with little or no results.

We, however, will tell you as accurately as possible all the information you need to know concerning your body as it relates to achieving fitness. We also will tell you how to achieve the positive results that you desire with a program that is personally yours. Hopefully, after completing this book, you will want to be physically active in some way. It *is* possible to find an activity or two which you really can enjoy and can participate in to the degree that you can achieve and maintain a reasonably fit body.

The definite advantages for women of some type of physical activity is constantly supported by published research. Our hearts will function more efficiently, we will maintain flexibility over a longer period of time, we can deal with stress better, we can control our weight, and we generally will feel better. With

1

this in mind, if you want to know about fitness and how to get started on an exercise or activity program, this book is for you. Even if you really hate physical activity, we urge you to read this book before you totally disregard participating in a sport or activity. With all the activities available today, surely there is something that will appeal to you.

BENEFITS OF BEING FIT

To exercise for the sole purpose of living longer may be important to some people. However, we believe that the benefits received from some form of physical activity not only can be long-term but can be gained as soon as you begin your fitness program and as you progress to a level at which your total physical and mental well-being are in harmony.

Women who currently participate in some type of activity will tell you from their own experiences with fitness programs that you not only will look better but you will feel better. You are better able to handle stressful situations. Your mental capabilities improve. You will find that you can concentrate better and for a longer period of time. The mind and the body cannot be separated, and as your physical well-being improves, so does your mental well-being. Thousands of women of all ages are turning to some form of physical activity because other women have told them how it has improved their lives.

A regular fitness program can, indeed, benefit you by helping you control your weight. As you grow older, your physical activity and metabolic rate (the rate at which the body uses energy and nutrients from foods) decrease, yet your food intake tends to remain about the same. This is when fat starts to accumulate in certain areas of the body, depending upon your particular body structure and genetic endowment, and you begin to see changes in the way your clothes fit and in your physical inability to do many activities that you were able to do when you were younger.

For women past age 25, watching what is eaten is a *must*. This is the approximate age when women should reduce the amount of food they eat because their amount of physical activity and their metabolic rate decrease. To maintain weight you must balance your intake (food) with your outgo (activity). If you want to lose weight, your activity must increase or your food intake must decrease. Physicians, physical educators, and others associated with weight control advocate a sound diet combined with a regular exercise program for maintaining proper weight.

As a result of maintaining your proper weight, your clothes will fit better. Although your weight may not change initially, you will find a change in inches in parts of your body. This is because you are replacing the fat with muscle, which weighs more than fat. Once you achieve good muscle tone the fat stores will start to disappear and weight loss will begin to occur.

In a more specific sense, physical activity can increase your physiological capabilities, that is, increase your strength, endurance, and flexibility for all tasks. With these assets come decreased incidence of low back pain, increased muscle strength to protect bones from breaking, and increased efficiency not only in normal daily tasks but in tasks required in emergency situations.

Another aspect of physical activity is your self-esteem and self-concept. You become more aware of your body and muscles and what they can do. You will be surprised at your capabilities, and accompanying that surprise will come the realization that you are capable of many things you once thought impossible. If you never have run a mile before and you finally accomplish this feat, or if you swim a quarter of a mile without stopping, the result is a marvelous feeling inside that you did it all by yourself. Your self-esteem will rise dramatically.

Although physical activity has many claims, we must acknowledge the fact that it *may* increase your life span and it *may* decrease certain physiological changes with age. We do believe, however, that regular physical activity will increase the quality of your life.

WHAT IS FITNESS?

Physical fitness is defined by the experts as the ability to carry on everyday activities without undue stress or fatigue and to be able to meet emergencies should they arise. This means that the degree of fitness varies among people according to the amount of activity in which they are involved. So, the concept of being physically fit will be different for everyone. This is important to remember. The degree of fitness fluctuates in each individual according to her state of health and ongoing activity.

Fitness is more than just being able to exist or survive. It is having the ability to pursue leisure activities as well as to engage in household chores without feeling out of breath, in pain, under stress, or totally exhausted in just a short period of time.

What all this means is that you should be physically active to the point where you feel good about yourself, your body, and your weight. You should have the energy to be able to do all the things you want to do. Of course, we cannot tell you that you *must* do this or you *must* do that. But, if you believe you should get more physical activity than you are getting now, the following chapters will provide some basic information about physical activity and then will present several alternatives toward obtaining fitness.

Hard Truths about Achieving Fitness

1. Fitness is not easy to achieve. You will have to work at it.
2. Once achieved, fitness is easier to maintain but you constantly must work at it.
3. Fitness cannot be achieved sitting down or lying down.
4. Fitness cannot be achieved in thirty minutes a week or in a few days. The worse shape you are in the longer it will take, from a period of a month or two to several months.
5. Fitness cannot be achieved by diet alone.
6. Fitness means you *will* perspire.
7. Fitness requires self-discipline. No one can make you do anything.

WHAT ARE THE COMPONENTS OF FITNESS?

There are three major components of fitness: muscular strength and endurance, flexibility, and cardiovascular endurance (aerobic capacity). In addition to these components, body composition is an important consideration because the amount of body fat you have will affect your overall abilities.

Muscular Strength and Endurance

When people talk about strength, they generally are talking about muscular endurance or the number of times they can repeat an exercise. Strength, by definition, is *one* all-out effort by a muscle or muscle group. For example, if you can do one push-up, you are displaying strength of your shoulder girdle and arm muscles. If you can do more than one push-up, you are showing that those muscles have endurance or the ability to repeat the exercise.

Muscular strength and muscular endurance are specific to the muscle or muscle group on which you work. They also are specific to the angle at which you work. For example, if you work your biceps with the arm bent at 90 degrees, your biceps will be strong at 90 degrees but not at any other angle. Strength training should be done throughout the range of motion of the joint so that you can be strong in any position.

Although little is known concerning the physiological aspects of strength gain, we do know that strength is an important component for fitness. Many women refrain from engaging in strength training for fear of getting bulging muscles (hypertrophy). Consequently, their leisure-time activities suffer because strength is such a vital component to adequate participation in all physical activities. Evidence has shown that women can increase their strength yet not obtain bulging muscles because women do not have the abundance of the hormone testosterone, which is believed to cause muscle definition.

Today, most strength training is called weight training and is done on some type of gym equipment, such as the Universal Gym (Fig. 1), Nautilus equipment (Fig. 2), or free weights (barbells) (Fig. 3). There are three terms connected with strength training: isometrics, isotonics, and isokinetics.

Isometrics are exercises that are done against a resistance that will not move. For example, pushing the palms of your hands together is an isometric exercise for the chest muscles (pectorals) (Fig. 4). The chest muscles are contracting yet no movement of the body takes place. Voluntarily contracting your stomach muscles is another example of isometric exercising.

Isotonic exercises are exercises that involve movement of the body or parts of the body when the muscle or muscle group

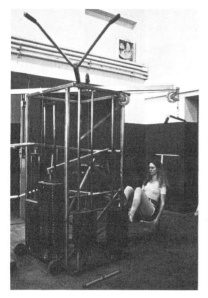 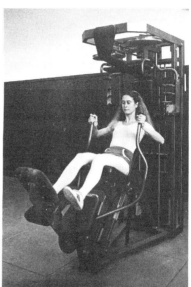

Fig. 1 Universal Gym   *Fig. 2 Nautilus equipment*

contracts (Fig. 5). Almost everything we do is isotonic: stooping, lifting, walking, sit-ups, and so forth. The term isotonics, however, is most often referred to as exercises done on gym equipment.

The Nautilus and Universal equipment designers have developed a technique with their machines called "variable resistance." When you lift a weight, the hardest part is getting started. Once the weight is moving it is easier to keep lifting it. Because it gets easier, you are not getting the overload placed on your muscles that you need in order to build strength. The accommodating resistance effect of the weight-lifting machines apparently corrects for this lack of overload by keeping the weight at a maximum at all times throughout the movement.

Isokinetic exercises vary from isotonic exercises in that they have accommodating resistance throughout the range of motion of the joint. That is, the resistance is adjusted to the movement so that maximum force must be exerted throughout the movement, and the speed of the movement remains constant. Only one isokinetic machine exists today, and it is used primarily in rehabilitation centers (Fig. 6).

Flexibility

The second component of fitness, flexibility, means the ability of each joint to flex (bend) and extend (straighten) throughout a wide range of motion. Flexibility, like strength, is joint-specific. Just because you do a backbend does not mean that you can do the splits.

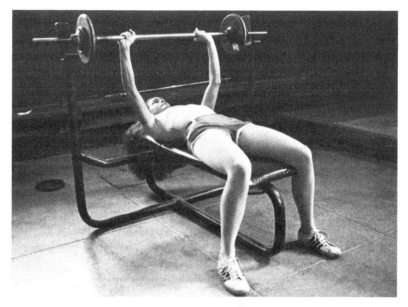

Fig. 3 Free weights

Some people who are very flexible in all their joints are commonly referred to as "double-jointed." However, there is no such thing as a double joint: the joint is either shallow or the ligaments are loose, which allows for this extra freedom of movement. People with loose ligaments need to work on maintaining strength in the surrounding musculature, which will help maintain the integrity of the joints and prevent injuries. They do not need to do an extensive number of flexibility exercises because a few repetitions are adequate.

Loss of flexibility seems to be a factor in the aging process, as witnessed by older people who have hunched shoulders and are generally stiff throughout their bodies. Maintaining flexibility should be focused upon by *all* adults to help retard the aging process.

Cardiovascular Endurance

Cardiovascular endurance, as opposed to muscular endurance, is related to the heart and its functioning ability. Cardiovascular endurance is the ability of the heart to pump blood to the lungs to get oxygen and then on to supply the muscles and tissues of the rest of the body. The common term used today for this component of fitness is "aerobics," or the use of oxygen while exercising. The better cardiovascular endurance an individual has, the more efficient her heart is. Running is the main activity that is popular today that builds cardiovascular endurance in a relatively short period of time.

Body Composition

A final consideration to overall fitness is body composition, which consists of the percentage of body fat in an individual, the weight of the fat, and the lean body weight. Recent evidence suggests that too much fat affects the physical fitness and health of an individual and, consequently, more attention must be paid to the percentage of body fat in our bodies. Ideally, women should have 16 to 20 percent of body fat; that is, 16 to 20 percent of a woman's total weight should be body fat. In reality, most women have between 25 and 30 percent body fat.

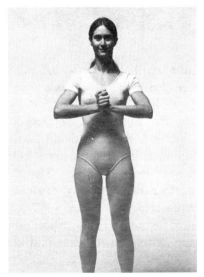

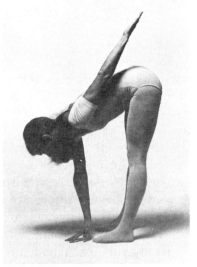

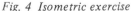

Fig. 4 Isometric exercise   *Fig. 5 Isotonic exercise*

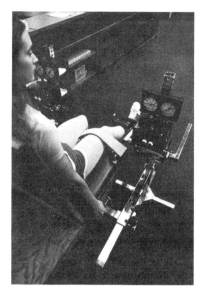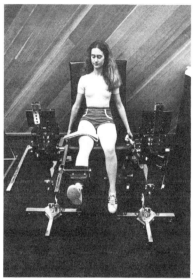

Fig. 6 Isokinetic machine

EVALUATING YOUR PRESENT FITNESS

Muscular strength and endurance, flexibility, cardiovascular endurance, and body composition are the four areas in which to determine your present fitness. Below are some simple tests to evaluate yourself. Do not attempt any of these tests if you have any type of physical problem such as a heart condition or joint problems. *Check with your doctor first.* Do not continue any of the tests if you feel strain or stress at any time.

Strength Tests

Try to perform one of each of the tests. If you can do at least *one* you have a good base on which to start your fitness program. If you cannot do each test, you should think seriously about establishing *your* fitness program.

1. Lying down on your back with your *legs bent*, feet flat on the floor, hands behind your head, leading with your head, curl up to a sitting position. Try to do this without someone holding your feet. This tests the strength of your stomach muscles. (See sit-up, p. 48.)

2. Lying face down on the floor, hands under your shoulders, toes curled under, body straight, perform one push-up so the arms are completely extended. Keep your entire body completely straight. This tests arm and shoulder girdle strength. (See push-up, p. 59.)

3. Grasp a bar with your hands and hang from it. Lift with your arms so that your chin comes above the bar, then lower yourself slowly. This is a test of arm strength. (See chin-up, p. 63.)

4. Lie facedown, hands behind head and someone holding your feet. Arch your back so that you lift your head and upper body off the floor. This is a test for back strength. (See back arch, p. 44.)

5. Standing with your back straight, bend your knees to at least a 90-degree angle (right angle) to your lower leg (but not all the way into a deep knee bend), and return to a standing position. This is a test for leg strength (Fig. 7).

Muscular Endurance Tests

Tests of muscular endurance include all of those mentioned for strength, but repeat them as many times as you can up to twenty times. If you can perform all of the strength tests twenty times you have good general body strength and ought to remain that way. If you have access to barbells or weight machines, you can perform similar tests of strength by doing such exercises as the bench press, squats, overhead press, and the dead lift. Anyone who is unfamiliar with barbells or weight machines should consult a knowledgeable trainer to understand these exercises and to have them demonstrated before trying them herself.

Flexibility Tests

Tests for flexibility focus on the ability to flex and extend the joints.

1. Standing with legs straight, touch your toes. This tests back and leg flexibility.

2. Lying on your back, grasp one knee and lift your head to try to touch your forehead to that knee. Try the same thing with the other knee. This tests back flexibility. (See knee-to-nose touch, p. 44.)

3. Sitting or standing, reach over one shoulder with one arm, reach behind the back with the other arm, and try to grasp hands. Try this in both directions. This tests shoulder flexibility. (See back clasp, p. 40.)

4. In a standing position, put your toes on a two-inch board with your heels still on the floor. As the next step, stand up with your heels on the board and touch your toes to the ground. This tests ankle flexibility and calf flexibility (Fig. 8).

5. Stand about two feet from a wall and, with your body absolutely straight and your heels on the floor, lean to the wall. How far back can you move your feet from the wall and still keep your heels on the ground? Eighteen inches is good. This tests flexibility in the back of the leg and calf. (See calf stretch, p. 34.)

6. In a standing position, hold onto a doorknob or wall. Grasp one foot behind you and touch your seat with your heel without arching your back. Try this also with the other foot. This tests the flexibility of the front of the thigh. (See thigh stretch, p. 38.)

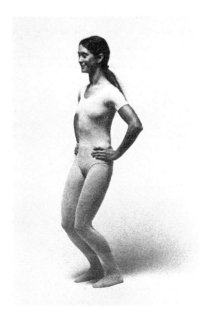
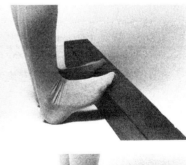
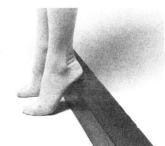

Fig. 7 Half knee bend   *Fig. 8 Toe and heel stretch*

7. Standing, with your feet shoulder-width apart, slide your right hand down the side of your leg as you bend to the right. Can you get your hand past your knee? Try this to the left side. This tests the flexibility of the sides of the body. (See side bends, p. 24.)

8. Lying face down, grasp both feet, head up. Can you arch your back enough so that you can rock back and forth on your abdomen? This tests the flexibility of your abdominal muscles and back. (See rocker, p. 36.)

If you can perform all of these exercises comfortably, you are flexible and you should keep up your present activity to maintain this flexibility. If you cannot do any one of the exercises, think about starting an activity program now!

Cardiovascular Tests

There are several cardiovascular tests that can measure the efficiency of your heart and lungs. The tests are best done in an exercise physiology laboratory, where you can either run on a treadmill or ride a bicycle while oxygen is collected from you.

There are some tests you can do outside the laboratory, but most of these involve special equipment. If you can run comfortably the best test is the one established for women by Cooper and Cooper in *The New Aerobics*. There is a specific scale for you to determine your fitness level according to how far you can run in 12 minutes.

If you want to test your cardiovascular efficiency and running is out of the question, the next best test you can do at home is a step test. Described below is a step test from which you can get some idea as to your level of cardiovascular fitness.

You will need a twelve-inch-high bench or step, a clock, and a metronome if you have one. Be sure to rest five minutes before the test, and don't eat or smoke at least one hour before the test.

First, record your resting heart rate to make sure you are truly rested (Fig. 9). Then, step for three minutes on the bench at a rate of twenty-four steps per minute (two full steps every five seconds, ninety-six total counts per minute). The sequence for one full step is: up right foot, up left foot, down right foot, down left foot. Keep your back straight.

When you complete your three-minute stepping, sit down and within five seconds take your heart rate for one full minute. Table 1 will help you determine your fitness level.

TABLE I
FITNESS LEVEL STANDARDS FOR KATCH STEP TEST

	30	30-39	40-49	50-59	60+
Excellent	0- 80	0- 82	0- 84	0- 90	0- 98
Very Good	81- 88	83- 92	85- 93	91- 99	99-108
Average	89-102	93-106	94-108	100-114	109-124
Below Average	103-110	107-115	109-117	115-123	125-134
Poor	111-	116-	118-	124-	135-

(Age)

Body Composition

Your main concern is the percentage of your weight that is body fat. There are two tests you can do at home to determine your body composition. Keep in mind that accurate body composition results can be obtained only through laboratory methods (total skin fold measurements with calipers or underwater weighing in a tank).

Look at your entire body in the mirror, front and back. How does it look to you? Do you see fatty areas that weren't there when you were younger and shouldn't be there now?

Next, grasp the skin behind your upper arm with your thumb and forefinger (Fig. 10). If the thickness is greater than one inch (from thumb to forefinger), you have too much body fat. One of the primary fat deposit sites is behind the upper arm, so although this test is very rough, it will give you an idea about your overall body composition. (Other fat deposit sites are the stomach and thigh.)

Now you should have an overall picture of your present fitness level. If you can perform and pass all of the previous exercises and tests, congratulations and keep up the good work. If you

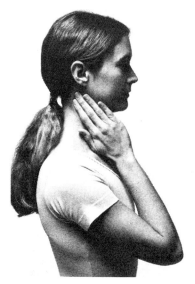

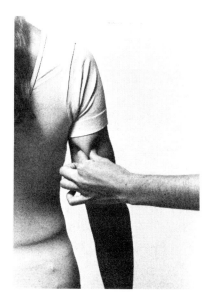

Fig. 9 Pulse check   Fig. 10 Pinch test

could not pass some of the tests or did not do well, think seriously about getting involved in some sort of fitness program. Remember that you must work in all the areas: flexibility, strength, and cardiovascular endurance. These are the areas necessary for achieving fitness. Your body composition will be affected by participation in these three areas.

One final point that should be made is important, true, and not very pleasant. Engaging in physical activity is not easy, nor is it always a pleasure to do. Staying in shape requires effort on your part because no one else can do it for you.

The benefits of exercise far outweigh the uncomfortable times when every step or movement seems like an ordeal.

So don't be dismayed. We all have our bad days when we don't feel like exercising. That's all right. Don't constantly force yourself to do something you truly dislike. Find an activity you like to do *most of the time* so that the good times you have participating in that activity will help you get through the hard times. Many people are *enjoying* physical activity these days and you can too. It is worth thinking about it and doing it as well.

2

Information For Your Fitness Program

Now you have a basic understanding of what fitness is all about. You also have a good idea about your own fitness level as well. Remember, you want to achieve the best physical condition *within your own body structure*. The following basic information should be adhered to in your activity program.

Rules for Safety

If you arc more than thirty years old and have not had a good physical examination by a physician within the past year, you should get one. Tell your doctor that you plan to take part in a fitness program of some kind and ask if you have any limitations. If you know what your fitness program will be, tell your doctor and make sure there will be no problems before you begin. If you are younger than thirty and are healthy, you should be able to participate in any type of activity if you make sure your program is gradual and sensible. If any abnormalities occur, visit a physician.

Find an activity that you truly enjoy and participate in it with as much gusto as possible. You should not continue with the activity, however, if any undue stress or pain occurs. Any activity, in order to be effective, will have some amount of stress and pain associated with it, but there is a line drawn between when the stress is good for you and when it will cause harm. If you are not sure about a particular stress or pain you experience, ask a reliable person, such as a coach of that activity, a physical educator, a physician, or someone who has participated in that activity for a while. Explain your symptoms and find out if they require special attention. It is wise to ask someone before beginning the activity what to expect so that you will be psychologically prepared beforehand.

When you engage in any activity, try to become active enough to get your heart rate up to about 70 percent of your maximum heart rate. To determine this, subtract your age from 220 and then take 70 percent of that number. The resulting figure is where your heart rate should be for a "training effect" to occur.

For example, if you are forty years old, subtract forty from 220. Multiply that number (180) by 70 percent and you get 126. Your heart rate, then, should be around 126 beats a minute for the activity to have its most beneficial effect on your body.

One of the purposes of exercise is to improve your present fitness level and to do this you must work hard enough to get a training effect. That is, you are exerting enough effort to make your heart beat at least 70 percent of maximum, and this will in turn increase the total efficiency of your body. Another way to look at this is to apply the "overload principle" to any activity in which you participate. Do the activity until you feel tired and then do it a little bit longer. If you do this each time you are active, you will be able to participate longer and longer and with more efficiency.

Whatever activity or exercise program you participate in, make your program progressive. Don't start off with hard exercises or strenuous activity. Instead, work up to the hard parts gradually. It may be frustrating at first because you will want to push yourself, but pushing won't work. Injuries could result and then you would be worse off than when you began. Don't be impatient. It will take *at least a month* for your body to become adjusted to the physical activity if you haven't done anything in a long time.

Be sure to acclimatize to any different environment in which you exercise. If you travel a lot, find out what the humidity and altitude are and take things slowly at first. This won't be true for just an exercise program but it will be for any other type of activity such as golf, tennis, racquetball, bicycling, or running.

Don't forget to breathe when you exercise or do any type of activity. Many people hold their breath when they exercise and then they wonder why they get dizzy or feel bad. Remember that your muscles need oxygen to work and the only way they get oxygen is by your breathing.

When doing basic exercises or exercises on machines, any movement done slowly with heavy resistance will tend to cause enlargement of the muscle (hypertrophy). If you exercise rapidly with a light resistance you tend to reduce that area. (Actually, the muscles you exercise at a fast rate of speed probably remain the same size—it's the fat stores that are being used up.) If you want to round out your figure or "shape up," you can adjust your exercises by altering the resistance and the speed of movement.

For example, let's say you would like the calves of your legs larger but your thighs smaller. You can hold weights in your hands and do toe raises several times for calf development, but you can do side and front leg lifts quickly with no resistance for your thighs to get smaller. In any case, it is best to do all exercises at a moderate speed.

Always do some basic stretching (flexibility) exercises before and after *any* type of activity. This will warm up your muscles and prevent injuries.

Clothing

There is a wide variety of clothing on the market to wear for the many sporting activities. The main items you see advertised are jogging clothes, tennis wear, and leotards.

Two things should be considered when buying exercise clothes. First, make sure they are comfortable *everywhere* on you and that you can move freely. Second, try to get a material that is part cotton, preferably at least 50 percent. All-polyester outfits, although very stylish and good looking, are not functional as far as getting rid of heat because polyester does not absorb perspiration as cotton does. When cotton clothing gets wet, the surrounding air evaporates the moisture and cools the body. Little evaporation takes place under polyester clothes and so the body temperature tends to rise.

The same thing happens to nylon, but the nylon jogging

shorts currently in use are small enough not to be detrimental. (In high temperatures, heat exhaustion may occur. This is discussed in a later chapter.)

Wear shoes that are appropriate to the activity. Running shoes are made for running so don't use them for tennis or racquetball. Make sure the shoes fit properly. It is worth the money to invest in a good pair. Your feet take enough of a beating as it is, so, if you engage in an activity that requires being on your feet, good shoes are a must.

Wear a good support bra. We have found (through film analysis) that the larger a woman's breasts, the more force there is on them, which can lead to sagging as she gets older. Many of the bras on the market today offer poor support for any type of physical activity. Find one that fits snugly and holds you firmly when you run, jump, and so on. Get a special bra and keep it as your "sport bra."

Because of our study, many bra companies are now in the process of developing a good support bra for women who participate in physical activity. We hope, in the near future, that all women, regardless of size, will be able to find a good support bra in the stores and will feel comfortable while being active.

Equipment

Don't skimp on equipment! Our advice to all of you is to get the best equipment you can. That doesn't mean that if you play tennis you have to go out and buy a new $250 graphite racquet. Rather, don't go to your local discount store and buy a $1.98 racquet.

For the most part, you get what you pay for in equipment. Go to your local sporting goods store and ask the salesperson what is best for you at your skill level. If you can, check with more than one store before you buy. If you get good quality equipment to start with, two things will occur. First, you cannot blame your skill on the equipment. Second, since you've invested so much money in the equipment, you might feel guilty not using it—so you will use it more.

Duration

Many people ask, "How long should I exercise?" or "How many times a week should I exercise?" Scientific evidence has shown that if you exercise or participate in an activity, you can do it for a minimum of three days a week and still get effective results. So, whether you do it five, six, or three times a week doesn't seem to make a difference. If you can fit only three times a week into your schedule, try to spread it out over the week rather than cramming it all into the weekend.

When you are active, you should maintain a 70 percent heart rate for at least thirty minutes. That means that if you are doing strictly exercises, you must do the exercises at a good pace and move quickly from one to the other. Check your heart rate periodically to make sure it is in the right range for the training effect.

Certain sports, such as running, are better at maintaining the heart rate in the 70 percent range. Other sports, such as tennis, are more sporadic, so, if you engage in such activities, you'll have to participate longer than thirty minutes to get the same effect.

One of the reasons many people have turned to jogging as a method of exercise is that they can get their heart rates up, maintain them at 70 percent of maximum for thirty minutes, and then their exercising for the day is over. Plus, it takes little equipment and no special place to run.

Just remember, the less stress the activity places on your heart and muscles, the longer the period of activity will have to be in order to be effective for achieving fitness.

Location

The physical location of your activity program is important. If you do not feel comfortable where you are, you won't participate to your fullest. Let's begin with a basic exercise program.

One good thing about a basic exercise program is that you can participate almost anywhere. Wherever you can find a space to lie down and move about, approximately six feet square, will do. You'll need a high ceiling if you are going to jump rope, but other than that you can find some space in your own home to do your basic exercises. Try out different areas or rooms in your home to find the best location for you. Once you find the "spot," stick with it. It's easier to get in the habit of exercising when you have a spot primarily for that.

If you want to play tennis, racquetball, golf, and so forth, you have another problem. Hopefully, your town or city has a park nearby where tennis courts are available. Many times you will have to call in advance for reservations. This means planning your activity ahead of time, which has advantages and disadvantages. One advantage is that you tend to keep that reservation so you will participate in your activity. But a disadvantage is that you tend to put off making the reservation so you never can get a court available. This will take some organized, disciplined effort on your part.

If you belong to a health club or fitness center, you probably have to get in your car and drive there. This is another stumbling block, because you come home from work or your husband comes home from work and something always seems to come up and you "just can't make it tonight." Regardless of this, there usually are health clubs and fitness centers available for everyone.

Many communities have fitness programs through their local recreation centers or YMCA/YWCAs. These generally are good programs but they usually don't meet frequently enough for you to get fit. However, many times the things you do in these programs can be done at home, so you can get in your extra exercise days at home. Check your local universities and schools, too, because many times they have fitness programs during the week and ordinarily have excellent facilities.

Training Regimens or Programs

It is important to participate in a routine, whatever it may be, with your exercise program. If you are developing your own program, write it down on paper so you won't forget it and so you can follow it. Writing it down also will help you figure out if it progresses correctly and is suitable for you. Obviously, for tennis or other types of sports this is not necessary, but for exercise programs or fitness center programs, writing down your program can be helpful. (Fitness centers usually have set programs or make them out specifically for you.)

In any case, a training regimen will mean that you set aside a certain time regularly (three days a week, daily, or whatever) to engage in your activity program, and whatever that program is, you will stick to it.

3

Basic Exercises

There are numerous exercises for all parts of the body. We have selected several kinds of exercises that you can do in your home or in a gym. They are listed by categories of flexibility, muscular strength and endurance, and cardiovascular endurance. (Those exercises marked with an asterisk are good choices for a beginning exercise program.)

There are some points to mention first. DO NOT bounce in any of the flexibility (stretching) exercises. You set off a reflex action of the muscles to tighten when you want them to stretch instead. If you stretch slowly and do not bounce, you "sneak by" this reflex action and stretch the muscles without harming them.

Regardless of what exercises you do, there are certain parts of the body that won't respond as well as others to the exercises. This is because of the way in which you are built, not because the exercises are poor. For instance, the bulge of fat many women have on the inside and outside of the thighs is the hardest to get rid of and usually is inherited. The inside of the thigh is the hardest place to reach through exercise, and in general, spot-reducing exercises do not work.

When you exercise, you will lose fat in the areas where the concentration of fat is the greatest, so any noticeable change will take some time—*it won't happen overnight.* If you have heavy thighs and really are interested in trimming them up, you

21

will have to put forth a great deal of effort with diet *and* exercise.

Many women's magazines include exercise sections. Sometimes these exercises do not do what they say they will do. If you aren't sure, check with someone who ought to know (physical educator, coach, or physician). Many times if you do the exercise you can feel if it is doing what it says it will do. Becoming aware of each part and how it works is a good way of learning about your body.

When we talk about exercises for building strength, this means the same thing as firming or toning that particular area. You are getting rid of the fat as the muscle gets stronger. When we talk about flexibility exercises, this means the same as stretching exercises.

Flexibility: Trunk Stretch*

1. **Starting position**. Stand with your feet together, stomach in, arms stretched overhead.
2. Reach to the sky with one hand and then the other.
3. Then, bend over and try to touch your toes.

Repetitions: Do this several times slowly and you will find that you can go farther every time.

Benefits: This stretches your trunk when you reach up and the backs of your legs when you try to touch your toes. Flexibility is gained in the back and legs.

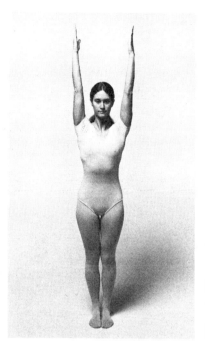
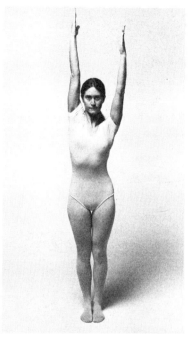
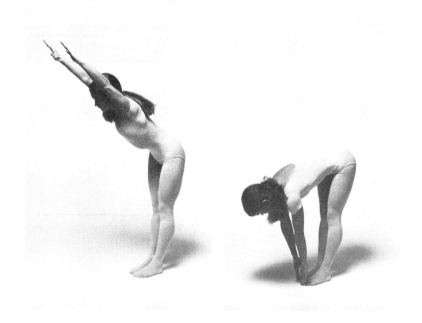

Flexibility: Side Bends*

1. **Starting position**. Stand with your feet apart, right arm above your head next to your ear and the left arm at your side.
2. Bend to the left, sliding your left arm down your leg, right arm still by your ear. Feel the pull on your right side as you do this.
3. Repeat this action to the right side, sliding your right arm down your leg, left arm by your ear. Feel the pull on your left side.

Repetitions: Do this **slowly**, twice on each side several times.

Benefits: Side bends are good for flexibility of the sides of the trunk.

Flexibility: Leg Stretch

1. **Starting position**. Sit with the bottoms of your feet touching each other.
2. Grasp your ankles and try to push your knees to the floor.

Repetitions: Repeat this several times.

Benefits: This is especially good for stretching the insides of the thighs, and increases flexibility of the hips.

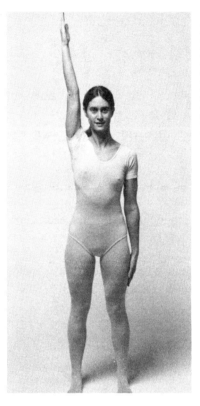
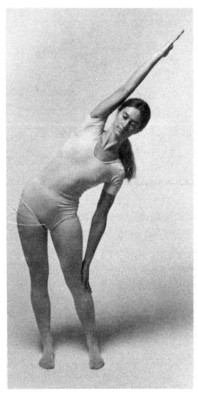
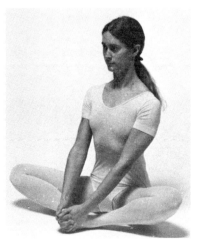
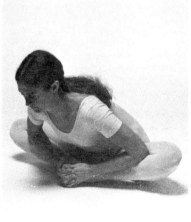

Flexibility: Leg and Trunk Stretch*

1. **Starting position:** Sit on the floor with your feet out in front of you.
2. Slowly grasp as far down your legs as you can with your hands and pull your upper body down, trying to touch your stomach to your thighs (top of head toward feet, keeping your legs straight).
3. When you get as far as you can, hold that position for a count of ten.

Repetitions: Repeat this several times, going farther each time. Remember to use a slow, steady pull. **Do not bounce.**

Benefits: The leg and trunk stretch increases flexibility in the back and legs.

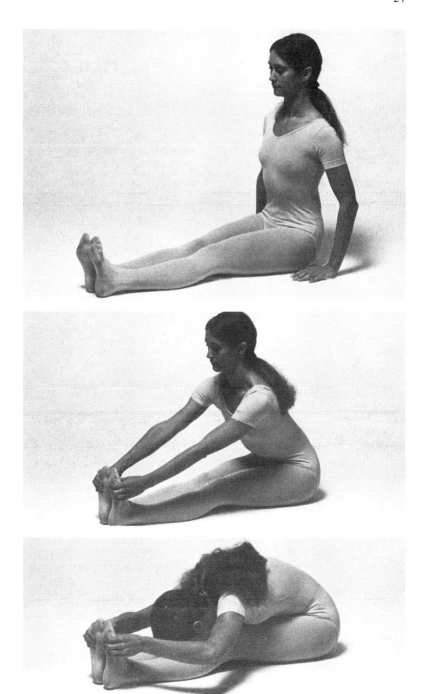

Flexibility: Leg and Trunk Stretch, Variation One*

1. **Starting position**. Same as basic leg and trunk stretch, but spread the feet apart.
2. Bend over one leg while grasping as far down that leg as possible and then over the other leg in the same way.

Repetitions: This should be done several times on each leg. **Do not bounce.**

Flexibility: Leg and Trunk Stretch, Variation Two (Hurdle Sit)*

1. **Starting position**. Sitting, extend one leg straight out in front of you but keep the other leg bent back and to the side.
2. Lean over the extended front leg as far as possible. Do not bounce.
3. Twist your body as far as it will go to the bent leg side.

Repetitions: Repeat on both sides.

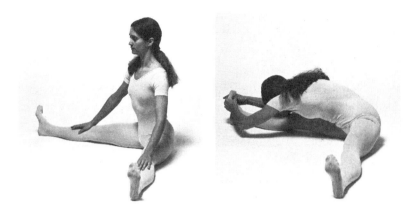

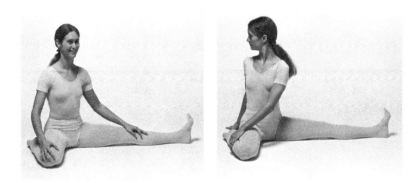

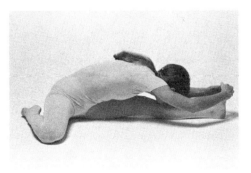

Flexibility: One-Half Backward Somersault

1. **Starting position.** Sit with your legs out in front, hands on floor at your hips.
2. Roll over backward, keeping your legs straight if you can.
3. Try to touch the floor behind you with your toes. (In yoga, this is called the Plough.) Hold this position for ten seconds.
4. Bend your knees and slowly roll to a sitting position.

Repetitions: Repeat this several times.

Benefits: This stretches the backs of your legs, your back, and your neck, encouraging flexibility in each.

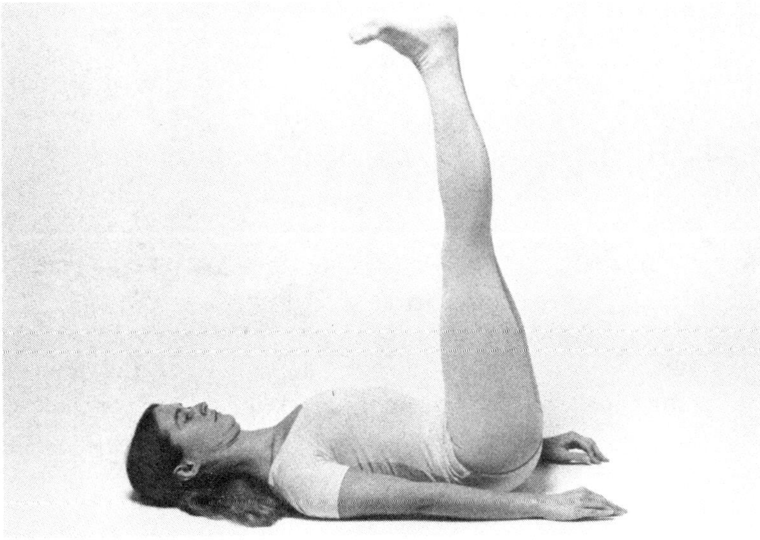

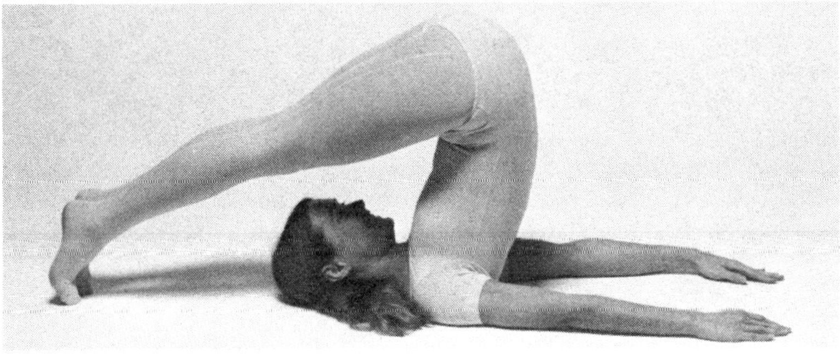

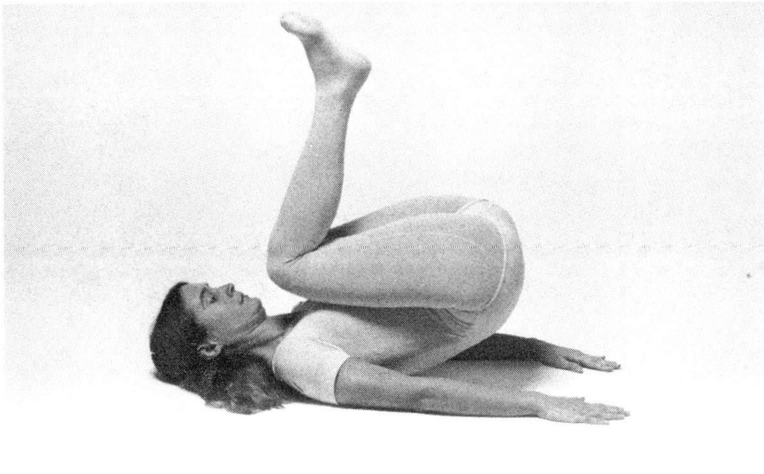

Flexibility: Side Leg Lifts*

1. **Starting position.** Lie on one side, using your top hand to prop yourself up so you won't fall over.
2. Lift the top leg without rotating it. (Do not point your toes upward. Keep the foot parallel to the floor.)

Repetitions: Repeat this fifteen times on each side at a moderate speed. Don't rush, and lift your leg as high as it will go.

Benefits: This exercise stretches the inside of the leg and strengthens the outside, prompting flexibility and strength in the hips and legs. If this is too easy for you, put on ski boots or hiking boots and do the same thing. This added weight will make it harder and more effective.

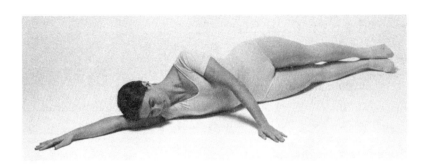

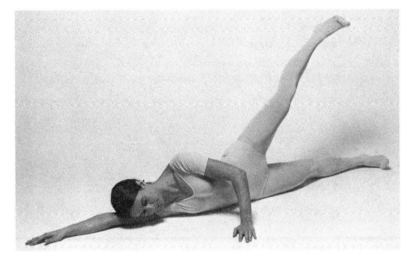

Flexibility: Calf Stretch

1. **Starting position.** Stand facing a wall (about two feet away) with your hands against it.
2. Keeping the body straight with heels on the floor, lean to the wall. **Your heels should remain flat on the floor.**

Repetitions: Hold this position for several seconds, rest, and repeat. If you do this easily, move farther away from the wall.

Benefits: The calf stretch creates flexibility of the calf.

Flexibility: Trunk Twists

1. **Starting position.** Stand comfortably, hands on your hips. (This is another exercise that can be done sitting at a desk.)
2. Twist the trunk twice in one direction and then twice in the other direction, going farther on the second twist.

Repetitions: Repeat this several times.

Benefits: Waist flexibility is maintained with this exercise.

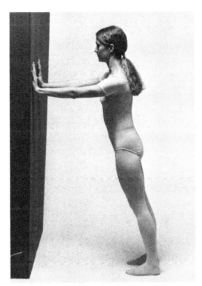 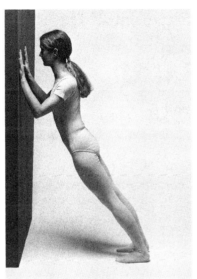

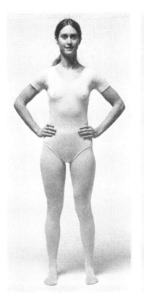 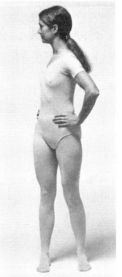 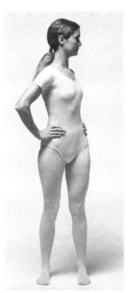

Flexibility: Head Roll*

1. **Starting position.** Sitting comfortably, concentrate on relaxing your shoulders. This can be done at a desk, in a plane, or anywhere.
2. Roll your head to the right a few times and to the left a few times. This should be done slowly.

Benefits: For flexibility of the neck and relaxation, the head roll is an ideal exercise. It gets the "kinks" out!

Flexibility: The Rocker

1. **Starting position.** Lying face down, bend your knees and grasp both ankles.
2. Pull your legs up as much as you can.
3. In this position, see if you can rock on your stomach.

Benefits: This exercise stretches the stomach muscles, promoting flexibility of these muscles, and helps strengthen the back muscles.

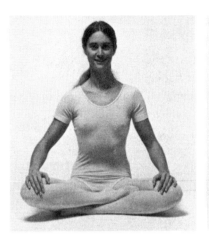
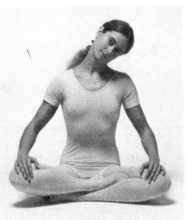

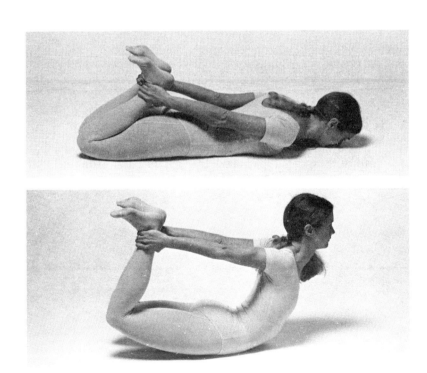

Flexibility: Back Reach

1. **Starting position.** Stand comfortably.
2. Grasp both hands behind your back.
3. Keeping your arms straight, bend over and try to put your hands over your head.
4. Go as far as you can, hold that position, and then rest.

Repetitions: Repeat periodically throughout your exercise period.

Benefits: This is good for stretching the front of your chest and shoulder muscles, and tightening the upper part of your back. It gives flexibility to the shoulders.

Flexibility: Thigh Stretch*

1. **Starting position.** Grasp one foot behind you. (You may want to hold onto a chair or wall for balance.)
2. Try to touch your heel to your seat.
3. Pull back so that you feel the pull on the front of your thigh. Keep lower back straight. That is, don't arch your lower back.

Repetitions: Repeat this several times on each leg.

Benefits: As its name implies, the thigh stretch is for flexibility of the thigh.

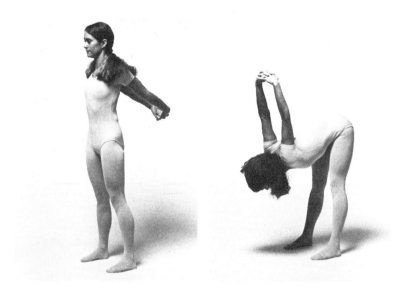

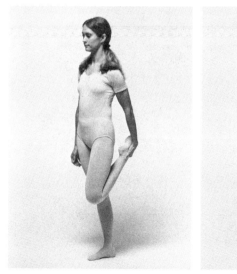

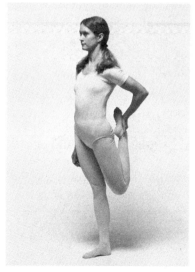

Flexibility: Arm Circles

1. **Starting position.** Stand comfortably with your arms straight out.
2. Rotate your arms in big circles both forward and then backward, keeping them straight. Concentrate on using your shoulders to do the work. (Do one arm at a time at first.)

Repetitions: Repeat ten times in each direction for each arm.

Benefits: Arm circles aid shoulder flexibility.

Flexibility: Back Clasp

1. **Starting position.** Sit or stand.
2. Put your right hand over your right shoulder and your left hand under your left arm—that is, behind you.
3. Try to grasp hands. If your hands don't quite reach each other, use a book, towel, or other object to clasp onto.
4. Try this on both sides.

Repetitions: This should be executed several times each day.

Benefits: This is a good test for flexibility of the shoulder area.

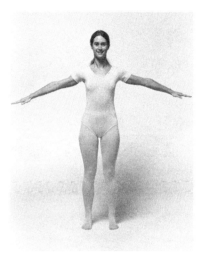
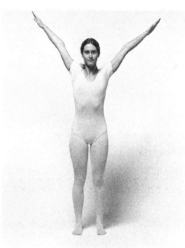
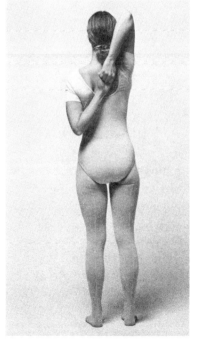
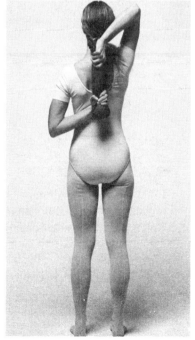

Flexibility: The Bicycle

1. **Starting position.** Lie on your back.
2. Roll back onto your shoulders, supporting your lower back with your hands.
3. Bicycle vigorously for fifteen seconds.

Benefits: This is good for warming up, loosening up the leg muscles, and getting the blood circulating. Flexibility, strength, and endurance of the legs and stomach result from this exercise.

Flexibility: The Bicycle, Variation One*

1. **Starting position.** Lower your hips to the floor from their position in the first bicycle exercise. Rest your arms on the floor, and keep your legs just above the floor.
2. Continue to bicycle for fifteen seconds.

Benefits: This bicycle requires more control than the basic bicycle exercise, and is good for the tops of the thighs and the stomach muscles.

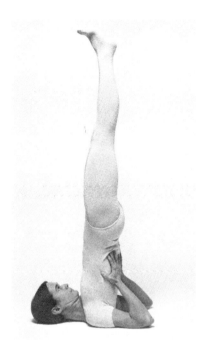
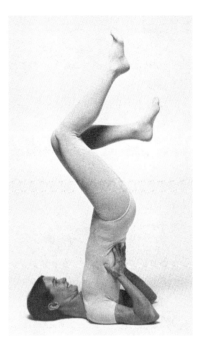

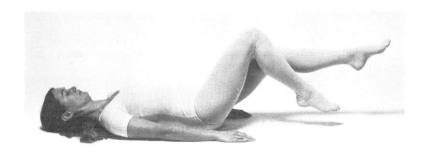

Flexibility: Knee-to-Nose Touch

1. **Starting position.** Lie on your back.
2. Grasp one knee.
3. Bring the knee to your nose, lifting your head up.
4. Try it with the other knee.

Repetitions: Repeat several times with each leg.

Benefits: A good exercise for stretching the back, neck, and seat, the knee-to-nose touch emphasizes flexibility of the neck and back.

Strength: Back Arch

1. **Starting position.** Lie facedown, hands behind your head. (You may need someone to hold your feet.)
2. Arch your back so that you lift your head and upper body off the floor.

Benefits: Back strength and endurance is built by the back arch. Do not do this exercise if you have low back pain problems.

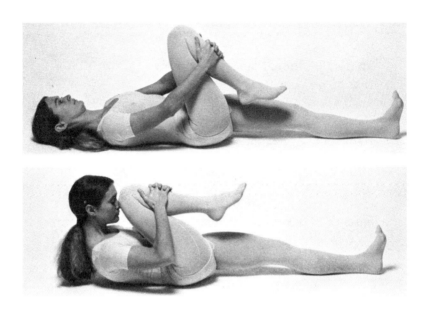

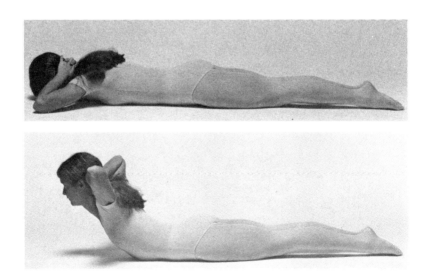

Strength: Leg Bends*

1. **Starting position**. Stand comfortably.
2. Rise up on your toes.
3. Bend your knees halfway.
4. Go back up on your toes.
5. Return to the starting position.

Repetitions: Repeat at least ten times, maintaining control.

Benefits: This is a great exercise for strengthening (and firming) the muscles of the entire leg and for building leg endurance.

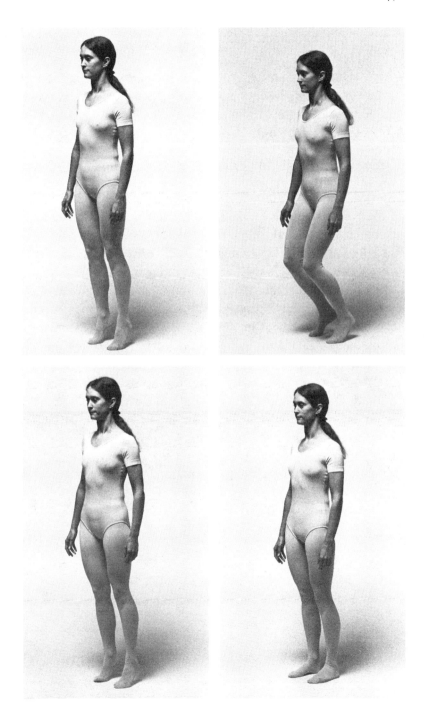

Strength: Bent Knee Sit-Ups*

1. **Starting position**. On your back, bend your knees and bring
   your feet as close to your buttocks as possible, hands behind your head.
2. Sit up.

Repetitions: Repeat as many times as you can, up to twenty
times.

Benefits: Bent knee sit-ups give strength and endurance to the
stomach muscles. If you lift only your head and shoulders off
the floor, you will be getting the same effect as if you did the
entire sit-up. Also, twisting your trunk as you sit up will use
more of your stomach muscles.

There are many variations of doing sit-ups, but the **knees
should always be bent in some way.** The knees are bent so that
the stomach muscles will do all the work, and so that the back
will not be strained.

When doing a sit-up with the legs straight, the lower back
muscles are used, especially one large muscle that goes from the
lower back over the pelvis to the top of the leg (the iliopsoas).
You do not want to use this muscle because it causes an arch
in the lower back where most low back pain occurs.

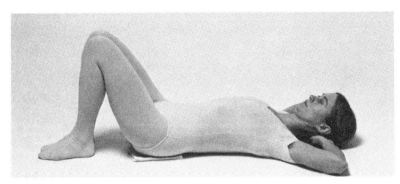

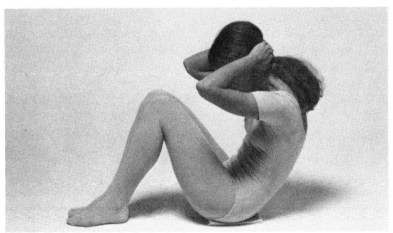

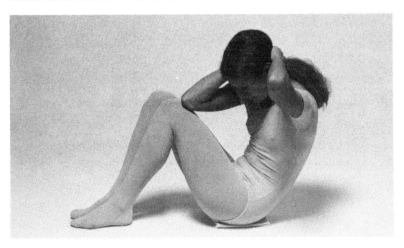

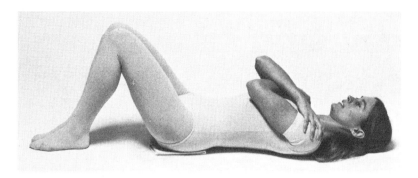

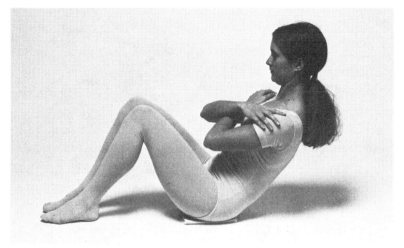

Strength: Bent Knee Sit-Ups, Variation One (Straight-Back Sit-Ups)

1. **Starting position.** Same as basic bent knee sit-ups, but with the hands crossed over the chest.
2. Sit up, keeping your back as straight as possible.

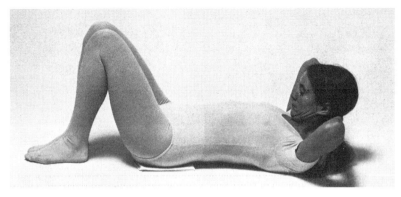

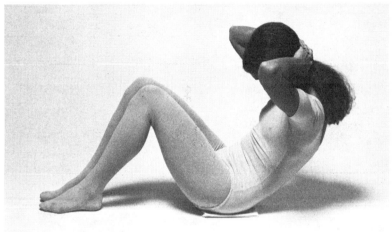

Strength: Bent Knee Sit-Ups, Variation Two (Curl-Ups)

1. **Starting position.** Same as basic bent knee sit-ups, but with chin on the chest.
2. Sit up with your back curled and with your chin remaining on your chest.

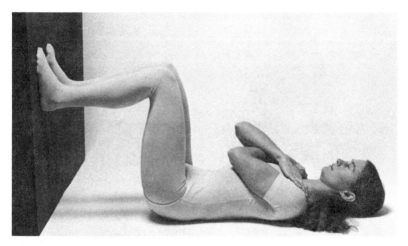

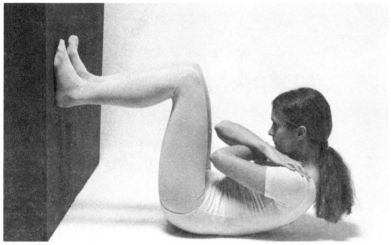

Strength: Bent-Knee Sit-Ups, Variation Three

1. **Starting position.** Lie on your back with your feet against a wall.
2. Sit up.

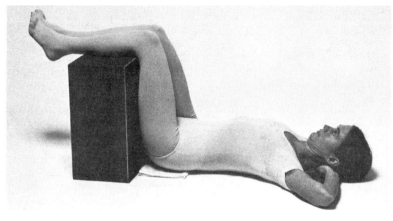

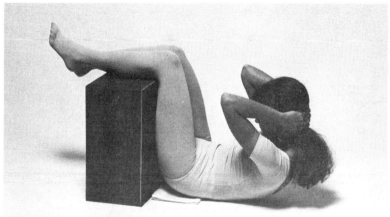

Strength: Bent Knee Sit-Ups, Variation Four

1. **Starting position.** Lie on your back with your feet over a chair.
2. Sit up.

Strength: Push-Ups* (Regular)

1. **Starting position.** Lie facedown on the floor, hands under your shoulders, feet together, toes curled under, body straight.
2. Push up so that your arms are completely extended. Keep your entire body completely straight.

Repetitions: Begin with one push-up, and gradually work up to ten, at which point you can level off.

Benefits: Push-ups build arm and shoulder girdle strength.

Strength: Push-Ups* (Modified)

1. **Starting position.** Same as in a regular push-up, except that you are on your knees.
2. Push up to full arm extension.

Repetitions: Begin with one and gradually work up to twenty, at which point you can level off.

Benefits: Again, a good exercise for building arm and shoulder girdle strength.

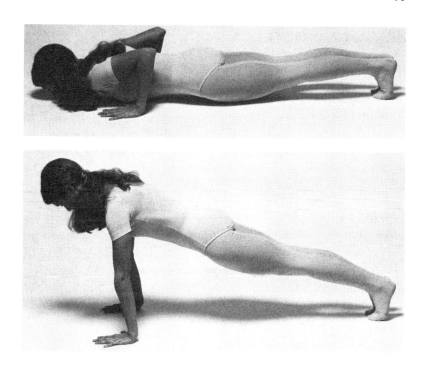

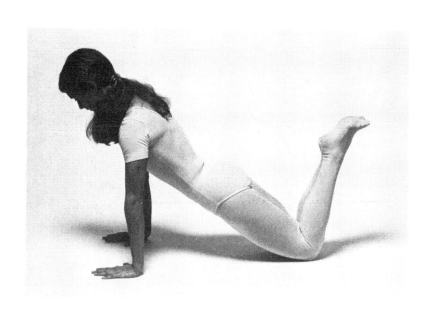

Strength: Push-Ups*
(The Wall Push-Off)

1. **Starting position.** Stand flat-footed about two feet from a wall, facing it.
2. Lean into the wall, keeping the legs and the entire body straight and the feet flat on the floor.
3. Push off from the wall until the arms are fully extended.
4. Lower yourself back into the wall.

Repetitions: Begin with one push-off and gradually build to twenty.

Benefits: As with the other variations of the push-up, the push-off builds arm and shoulder strength. In addition, it can be combined with the previously mentioned calf stretch to provide a good exercise for the upper body and lower legs.

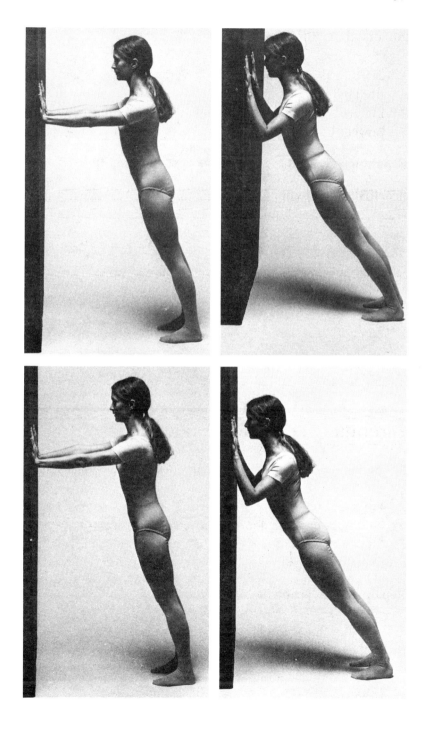

Strength: Chin-Ups

1. **Starting position**. Grasp a bar with your hands and hang from it.
2. Lift with your arms so that your chin comes above the bar.
3. Lower yourself slowly.

Repetitions: Repeat as many times as you can, up to ten.

Benefits: Chin-ups build arm strength.

Strength: The Pillow Squeeze

1. **Starting position**. Lie down or sit, knees bent, feet flat on the floor.
2. Put a big pillow or ball between your knees or make a fist with both hands and put it between your knees.
3. Squeeze your knees together as hard as you can for a count of ten.

Repetitions: Repeat this exercise ten times.

Benefits: The pillow squeeze helps firm the **inside** of your thighs.

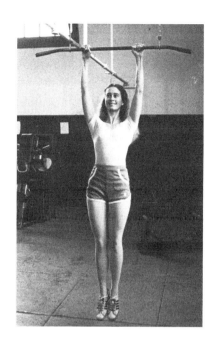

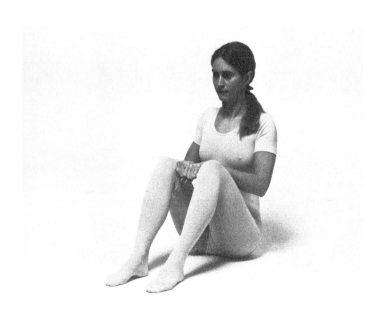

Strength: The Pelvic Tilt*

1. **Starting position.** Lie on your back with your knees bent.
2. Place your fingers under the small of your back.
3. Press your lower back into the floor so that you feel pressure on your fingers.
4. Hold this for a count of ten.

Repetitions: Repeat this action several times, trying to keep your pelvis "tucked in" at all times. Eventually do this without putting your fingers under your back.

Benefits: This is a good exercise for strengthening the lower back and for positioning the pelvis correctly so that backaches won't occur.

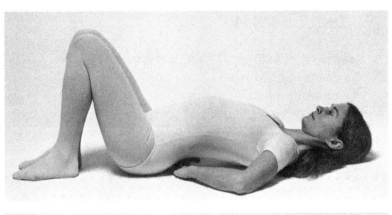

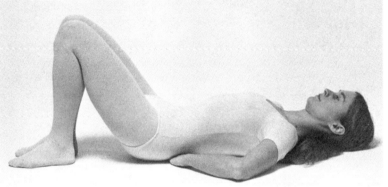

Strength: Leg Half Squats

1. **Starting position**. Stand with your feet wide apart.
2. Keeping your body erect, bend one leg partway.
3. Return to the starting position.
4. Bend the other leg halfway.

Repetitions: Repeat ten times to each side.

Benefits: These give strength and endurance to the legs, and firm up the thigh muscles. You might also want to try the half knee bend, pictured on page 11.

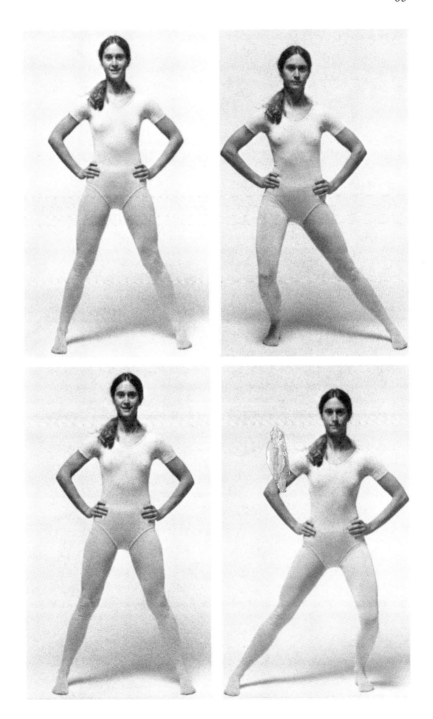

Strength: Rear Leg Lifts*

1. **Starting position**. Lie facedown, propped up by your elbows.
2. Lift one leg.
3. Lift the other leg. (Rotate each leg outward as you lift it.)
4. Then lift both legs at once.

Repetitions: Repeat ten times with each leg.

Benefits: This is a good exercise for firming up the back of the legs and your seat. It helps prevent a sagging bottom!

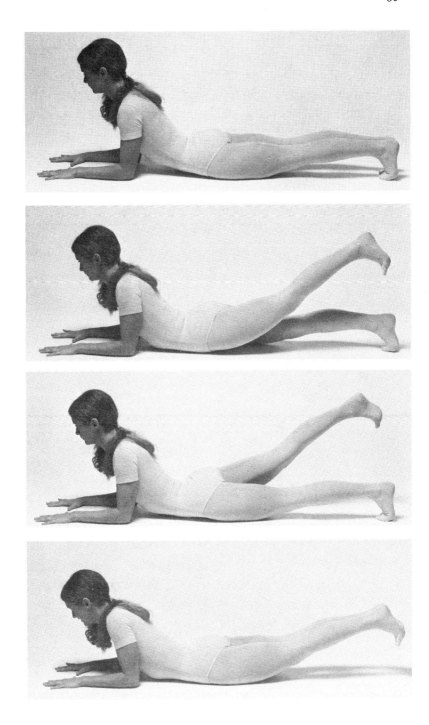

Cardiovascular Endurance: Jumping Rope

1. **Starting position**. Stand relaxed, keeping your grip on the handles and your wrists relaxed. Feet should be together.
2. Jump both feet at a time, springing only high enough to clear the rope. Land on the balls of your feet.

Repetitions: Start with jumping twenty times and increase the amount gradually.

Benefits: Jumping rope helps build strength of the legs and increases the functional capacity of the heart and lungs.

Cardiovascular Endurance: Jumping Rope, Variation One

1. **Starting position**. Same as the basic jump rope position mentioned previously.
2. Jump the rope one foot in front of the other.

Repetitions: Start with twenty and increase the amount gradually. Start working on speed, aiming for a slightly breathless state.

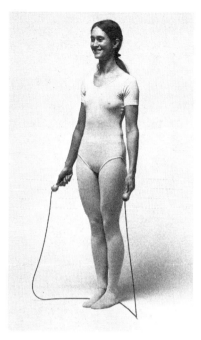
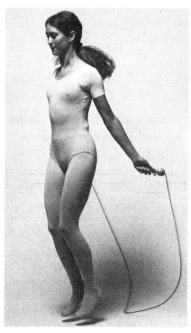
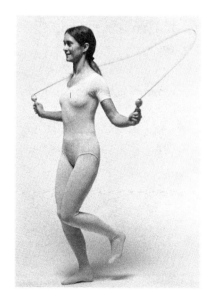

Cardiovascular Endurance: Running In Place*

1. **Starting position**. Assume a relaxed running position, standing straight, holding the head up and keeping the shoulders relaxed. Bend your arms about the waist high, and keep your hands cupped, not clenched.
2. Run for one minute at first, increasing the amount gradually.

Benefits: This is good for tightening the leg and stomach muscles, as well as building heart and lung capacity.

Cardiovascular Endurance: Running In Place, Variation One

1. **Starting position**. Same as the basic running in place position.
2. Run in place for one minute and then, for ten seconds, run while lifting your knees as high as you can.
3. Return to regular running. Gradually increase the duration of both types.

Waldenbooks

12 SALE 6879 0284/1 02/01/83

0890371636 4 1@ 4.95 4.95

SUBTOTAL 4.95
NEW YORK 7% TAX .35
TOTAL 5.30
PAYMENT 5.30

CHANGE .00

THANK YOU - PLEASE COME AGAIN

02/01/83 20:46

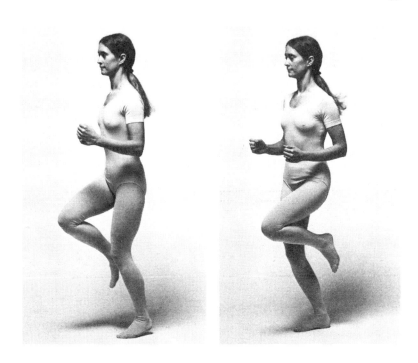

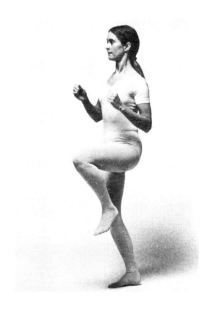

4

Fitness Activities

There are many different ways of achieving a fit body. All you have to do is pick a way (or several if you like) and stick with it. However, if you find that the activity you picked does not satisfy your needs, select another activity. As a matter of fact, it is nice to have two or three different activities that you can select. This will prevent you from getting bored with just one, and, hopefully, will keep you interested in obtaining and maintaining a certain fitness level.

Remember that different activities produce different fitness levels. For example, swimming laps thirty minutes every day will result in a more fit body than three hours of golf. It just depends upon what you want to do for your activity program. Very few activities have *all* the components of fitness (strength and endurance, flexibility, and cardiovascular endurance). In most programs you will need to supplement your primary activity with other activities or basic exercises such as those described in Chapter 3.

This chapter discusses all kinds of sports and activities and how their strengths and weaknesses relate to the components of fitness.

INDIVIDUAL ACTIVITIES

There are many individual activities that will help you achieve a fit body. Remember to warm up with some overall stretching exercises before any activity and to "cool down" with some after the activity is completed.

Walking

Walking is good exercise and cne which many people enjoy. To get any benefit from it, from a fitness standpoint, you should walk briskly. Try to walk a mile in fifteen minutes, being sure to maintain good posture (pelvis tucked in) and that you have on good walking shoes. Take good-sized strides and swing your arms freely as you walk.

Walk in areas where you don't have to look down at your feet, that is, where the sidewalks or streets are in good condition. Supplement walking with flexibility and strength exercises.

Yoga

Yoga exercises are excellent for stretching all parts of the body as well as for teaching control of the body. They can be done in your own home in a quiet, warm room. Ideally, you should do these exercises in the same place each time you exercise so that that place will hold some meaning for you.

Any book on yoga exercises will explain how to do them, or there may be courses on yoga available in your community recreation program. If you have never tried yoga, you should consider it if for no other reason than how terrific it makes you feel. For overall fitness achievement, however, it is necessary to do some other activity or exercise to strengthen your muscles and build cardiovascular endurance because yoga promotes neither.

Aerobic Dance

This is a form of exercise in which exercises and dance steps have been combined into routines and put to music. It is quite popular now and has many good points. It exercises all parts of your body and it works on all aspects of fitness: flexibility, strength, and cardiovascular endurance. Many routines have been devised, but you can make up your own. You will need a lot more space than for regular exercises and a record or tape player. With its increasing popularity, you can probably find a class in aerobic dance in your community.

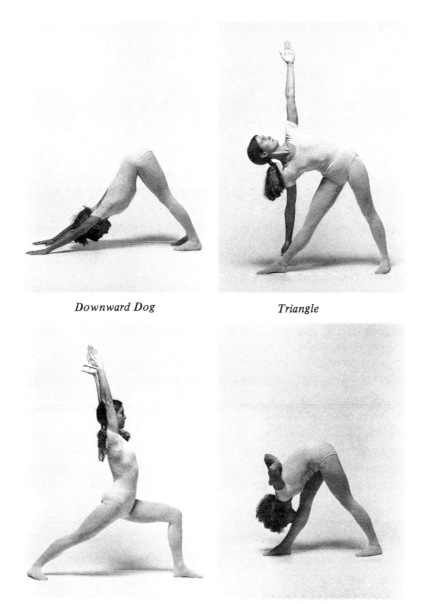

Downward Dog

Triangle

Warrior 1

Intense Side Stretch

Yoga Poses

Jogging or Running

As numerous books already written on the subject have suggested, jogging or running is a great activity for developing efficiency of the heart and lungs. You need little equipment, you do not have to have a special place to run, and you can get a maximum training effect in a short period of time. For a well-rounded activity program fulfilling all three components of fitness (muscle strength and endurance, flexibility, and cardiovascular endurance), you should supplement running with strength exercises for the upper body and flexibility exercises for the entire body.

There are those who hate the thought of running. It sounds boring or they cannot run because of physical problems. *Don't run if you do not like it!* But, by all means, give it a good try before deciding it's not for you.

Should you, in fact, decide to take up a running program, there are several ways of starting. (For details, you should refer to one of the many running books now available.) The main idea is to *start slowly*. Slowly build up your endurance and conditioning level.

With this kind of careful start, building a good base, you will be very pleased with your progress, and you will be much more apt to persevere. Basically, it is a matter of finding what is comfortable for you and then sticking with it. Commitment to a *regular* program of running slowly builds up your general physical endurance and conditioning. As you progress, it becomes easier, and you will begin to notice some interesting and enjoyable side effects.

Some authorities have suggested that the best measuring reference for beginners just starting a running program is time rather than distance. On different days you could run a significantly different amount of distance in the same amount of time, depending on how you feel, the weather, and other circumstances. Running a certain amount of time, therefore, may not be as discouraging a goal to the beginner as trying to run a certain number of miles each time out.

A good time goal to start with, according to some women runners, is thirty minutes. You can run slowly the entire time, or combine running with walking. Alternate the two and you will be surprised how quickly your body adapts. The main thing is to stick to a definite period of time, every other day, three to four times a week. This allows your body to adapt to the stresses of running gradually, with less risk of injury.

In the beginning, running is a stress because it is a new program of strenuous activity. As such, the first weeks of beginning running are not always pleasant. In the process of building a habit of this cardiovascular exercise, you can expect temporary aches and pains. Just remember that some women adapt to running more quickly than others, and age is not so much of a factor as the woman's basic level of physical capabilities.

As with any fitness program, learn to listen to your body. Before and after each run, warm up with stretching exercises. Run at a pace that allows normal conversation. Learn what time of day makes running easiest for you. Slowly increase your time (mileage) buildup after your first eight weeks of running. Include a longer run one day during the weekend, and then have a rest day. If you are running mainly for recreational purposes and to become more physically fit, then your goal does not need to exceed a maintenance level of forty minutes every other day, four days a week.

However, as you progress, suddenly feeling good and knowing your program is beginning to work, *take it easy.* If you suddenly increase your running time without allowing for adaptation, your body will respond with signs of overstress, such as fatigue, chronic aches and pains, colds, a desire for sweets, and sometimes even a feeling of depression or lethargy. You will be able to tell if you are adapting to running if you don't experience these definite signs of overstress.

Being aware of how your body is feeling helps lessen the chance of injury. Injuries in running are primarily caused by your body's reaction to overstress, so there is nothing wrong in cutting back your activity until the pain subsides. Pain merely is your body's way of telling you that something is wrong.

Women runners sometimes find their running to be a relaxing form of mental therapy as well as a method of physical fitness. Tensions at home or the office can be lessened by a relaxing run that leaves a feeling of invigoration. In addition, the time taken on a solo run allows time for yourself to think or just to let your mind wander.

Some women become almost dependent on running beyond diet or health reasons. They feel wrong if they miss a day of their schedule, running because they want to, not because they feel they "have" to. Others go on to become competitive racers. Whatever the motivation, running is an ongoing personal evaluation of exertion and satisfaction that has been enjoyed by many women as their main activity.

Archery

Archery coordinates the muscles of the back, shoulders, arms, and eyes, and is an excellent builder of poise and posture. It can be as leisurely or as competitive as one chooses, and interests both individuals and groups of all ages. Because a great amount of strength is not a prerequisite to success, women have been known to excel in this sport. Of course you will have to add activities to your fitness program that strengthen the lower body, stretch all parts of the body and encourage cardiovascular endurance.

Roller Skating

Roller skating develops balance, leg and arm coordination, basic body strength, good posture and, if done vigorously, it stimulates the cardiovascular system. An activity growing in popularity recently, it can be enjoyed indoors or out. Flexibility exercises, strength exercises, and stretching would have to supplement your skating, as well as another good cardiovascular activity.

Hiking and Backpacking

Backpacking has been valued by some as a fitness activity near to jogging in terms of energy consumed per number of miles covered, with day hikes with a light pack being one-half as beneficial as jogging. The amount of energy expended in mountain walking is substantial because of the added factors of the lower amounts of oxygen available at the higher elevations usually involved, and the extra quarter or so of your body weight on your back. Every time you gain a foot in elevation, you are lifting the total weight of your body and your pack that much.

To gain the necessary endurance to backpack in the thinner

mountain air and the necessary strength to carry added weight, jogging, brisk walking, strength exercises, and general flexibility exercises would be beneficial fitness supplements.

Bicycling

Bicycling is good cardiovascular training and excellent for leg strength and firmness, making it a good alternative to running. In addition, you don't have a constant beating of your feet and legs on the ground, so there are less physical (feet and knee) problems associated with bicycling.

Get a good bicycle that fits you properly, making sure the seat is adjusted for your leg length, and try to ride three miles in fifteen minutes in the beginning. You will have to ride longer than the thirty-minute requirement for the training effect to occur. Plot out several routes of various lengths in your neighborhood. Find out about bike safety rules and local laws. Many drivers resent bicyclists, so beware of cars and try to choose routes on side roads away from heavy traffic.

You will have to supplement bicycling with regular flexibility exercises for all parts of the body and some strength work for the upper body.

Water Sports

Kayaking, solo sailing, or solo canoeing are good activities for developing the upper body. If you live in an area where you have access to one of these water sports, try to take advantage of it. Again, you will have to supplement these activities with exercises for strengthening the lower parts of the body, stretching exercises for all parts of the body, and cardiovascular exercise.

Swimming

Swimming is the best all-around activity for all parts of your body *if* you use a variety of strokes, use correct form, and swim at a decent pace. In this activity, the upper and lower parts of the body move against a resistance (water), giving strength, and the rhythmic breathing works your lungs and heart. It also stretches many parts of the body, so there is some flexibility gained.

If you swim, it is best to swim laps. Try to swim for thirty minutes without stopping; it won't be hard if you intersperse the resting strokes with the harder strokes. Take your time, but keep going.

Some communities have "swimnastics" programs in which you do exercises in the water. This is fine, as it offers resistance to your movements and increases your strength, but that is about all it does. If you wish to pursue this activity, you'll have to supplement it with some activity that will increase your heart rate and breathing. You also will have to do some flexibility exercises out of the water to stay limber.

Skiing

Skiing falls into two categories: nordic and alpine. While nordic skiing (the cross-country type) is the more demanding on the body, both nordic and alpine rank high in all aspects of fitness. If you engage in either type, you will benefit.

The trouble with skiing is that most people do it only on weekends and do nothing during the week. It would be wise to engage in some other type of activity during the week, even if it is just basic exercises at home, to maintain a certain level of fitness for weekend skiing. There are many exercises and activities that complement skiing that you can do during the week, such as running, swimming, or tennis singles (to name a few). These would help you avoid fatigue and susceptibility to injury during those weekends when you are trying to ski as much as you can.

Skiing requires flexibility exercises for the whole body and upper body strength work as supplements.

Karate

Karate or any of the martial arts that are popular today require a great deal of effort and stamina, making them good activities for achieving a high level of fitness. There is plenty of flexibility and strength work, and the cardiovascular system is stressed, allowing a training effect to occur. This is an excellent activity for decreasing the size of the thighs—all that kicking really reduces those fatty areas on the thigh as well as on the whole body.

Ballet

Ballet is becoming a popular activity for women of all ages, and fortunately, dance studios and community recreation centers are now welcoming adult women.

Ballet requires discipline, and it is an excellent activity for developing flexibility and strength. However, it does not do much for cardiovascular fitness except on the advanced level, so you would have to supplement your ballet lessons with a cardiovascular activity such as running, swimming, or bicycling. (Assuming you have no major feet or knee problems, running is *not* detrimental to your performance in ballet.)

Horseback Riding

Horseback riding is the one sport that utilizes the inside of the thigh. (The exercise called "the pillow squeeze" is based on this principle.) Women who ride regularly have good strong thighs, especially on the inside.

Horseback riding demands leg strength and cardiovascular endurance, but you will have to supplement this activity with flexibility exercises for the whole body, strength exercises for the upper body, and, unless you ride long and hard, cardiovascular endurance exercises.

DUAL SPORTS

Dual sports are those activities such as golf, tennis, racquetball, or bowling, that involve more than one person but do not require a team.

Racquetball or Squash

The best dual sport for developing and maintaining fitness is racquetball or squash. The great amount of bodily movement in these sports gives a good workout for your heart and lungs, plus you build strength and endurance. The flexibility element is present, too, so all three components of fitness are involved in this activity. Extra flexibility exercises for all parts of the body are suggested as a supplement to this activity.

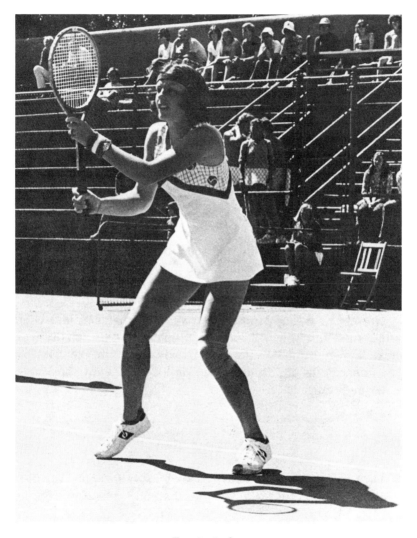

Tennis singles

Tennis

Tennis singles is better for developing fitness than doubles. If you have played both, you are aware that although the concentration is the same, you move a great deal more in singles. Also, in singles you move more consistently than in doubles, in which movement tends to happen in spurts. Tennis singles rates fairly high in all aspects of fitness but not as high as racquetball.

Badminton

Contrary to popular belief, badminton played as it was originally intended is a very vigorous activity. Most of us grew up learning backyard badminton, which is not as vigorous and the skill level of your teammates is usually not good. It is an excellent activity if played correctly because it demands cardiovascular endurance, strength, agility, and good reaction time.

Golf

Golf is much less strenuous and of absolutely no value for fitness if you take a golf cart. If, however, you walk *briskly* from hole to hole, you will increase your heart rate and the work of your lungs.

You have to have some strength and flexibility in your arms and shoulders to perform the strokes in golf, but not a great amount in other areas of your body. Supplemental work should be done in all areas of fitness for all parts of the body.

Bowling

Bowling is the least strenuous of this group of activities. It rates low in creation and maintenance of cardiovascular endurance, strength, and flexibility. If you like to bowl and do it frequently, that's fine, but you should supplement it with some cardiovascular activities for your heart and lungs plus strength and flexibility exercises or activities.

Fencing

Fencing develops coordination of mind and body while said to exercise every muscle of the body. The majority of fencers find fencing an excellent and interesting way in which to develop and maintain overall physical fitness. Success depends only on how each individual develops and employs her own particular physical predisposition. Relaxation, control, hand-eye coordination, and physical movements are only a few of the techniques taught.

At first, fencing may seem difficult and tiring. The physical movements and postures of fencing are not natural, so one needs to work toward strength gradually, until muscles have adjusted and developed to withstand the particular stresses imposed by the requirements of attack and defense movements. In a short time, however, the body strengthens and the mind adjusts to the uncommon speed of the activity. Many community recreation centers offer classes in this interesting sport.

Fencing should be supplemented by strength and flexibility exercises and a good cardiovascular endurance activity.

TEAM SPORTS

Team sports include soccer, basketball, softball, and volleyball. All team sports have periods of slow activity interspersed with periods of vigorous activity, so it is hard to rank any one as best in terms of fitness value. If you engage in these activities with as much vigor as possible to get your heart rate up and to breathe hard for a length of time, they are that much better for you. Don't forget to do warm-up and cool-down exercises (stretching exercises).

Basketball

Basketball can be a fast or a slow game. With teams comprised of five members in most areas of the country, basketball places more demand on the body than other sports and thus is better for obtaining fitness. If you play vigorously, you will be increasing your cardiovascular efficiency, your muscular strength, and, to a lesser degree, your flexibility. Many communities have basketball for women but generally the sport is played by younger women.

Soccer

Soccer is another sport attracting the attention of women that is a good activity for developing cardiovascular fitness, muscular strength and endurance, and flexibility. The forwards and halfbacks especially benefit in these areas, but other positions, such as the fullbacks, benefit to a lesser extent. The goalie has to be quick, agile, and strong enough to clear the ball, yet her heart and lungs are not being taxed at all. If you play a less vigorous position on a team, either try to alternate positions or supplement this sport with other more vigorous activities and exercises.

Volleyball

Volleyball can be a good activity for developing fitness depending upon how many people you have on a side. The fewer people there are on a side, the more strenuous the activity becomes and the better it is for developing fitness. This activity, like tennis, has spurts of vigorous movements and periods of mild movements. How active you are when you play will determine whether you need to supplement volleyball with another activity or exercise.

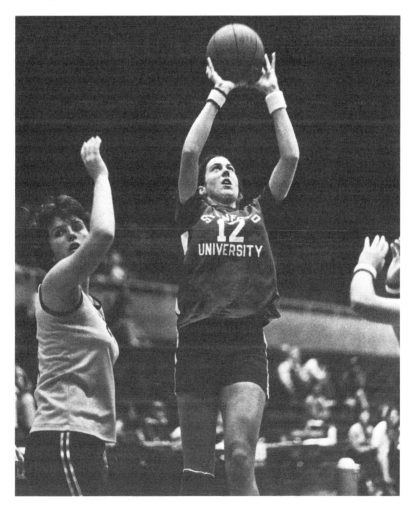

Basketball

Softball

Softball, both fast pitch and slow pitch, is another popular activity for women. The training appears to be more strenuous than the actual game, but you must have fast and strong legs with which to run the bases, and a strong arm with which to throw the ball. It is a good activity for muscular strength and endurance and to some extent flexibility, but very little stress is placed on the heart and lungs to develop cardiovascular endurance because you don't run long enough. You should supplement softball with flexibility exercises, strength exercises, and cardiovascular activities, which most coaches do in training programs.

Field Hockey

Field hockey is among the most popular outdoor sports played by women in this country. It is a primary school, secondary school, and college game, and many women continue to play throughout their adult lives. It is a challenging and exhausting activity that has been known as an exciting participatory and spectator sport.

Women's field hockey builds cardiovascular endurance and muscular strength. It should be supplemented with flexibility exercises.

WEIGHT TRAINING AND FITNESS CENTERS

Weight training for women is becoming very popular, especially now that women are realizing that they will not get bulging muscles if they train with weights. It is common today to see women training on all kinds of exercise machines who do not feel embarrassed or less feminine.

There are several kinds of equipment on which to train. Although athletes and coaches have "pet" ways to train, scientific evidence has shown that there is very little difference among the various methods of weight training.

Free Weights

The first kind of equipment is free weights, or what most would call barbells. They come both as dumbbells (Fig. 11) and as a bar on which you add "plates" (Fig. 3). If you plan to lift weights other than the little dumbbells, get instruction on how to lift the weights. This is very important because you could injure yourself if you lift them incorrectly.

Lifting free weights limits the areas of your body in which you can develop strength. You'll need to supplement this activity with flexibility and strength exercises in the areas not reached in lifting weights, as well as with some kind of cardiovascular activity.

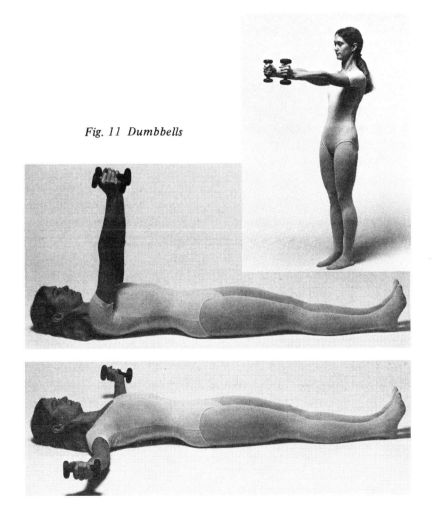

Fig. 11 Dumbbells

Universal Gym

The second piece of equipment is called the Universal Gym and is very popular with all athletic teams (see Fig. 1). This is a versatile piece of equipment in that it has something for every part of the body. You can establish your own level of fitness and work from there. Here is one workout you can do on this piece of equipment for each station.

1. Establish the weight you can lift ten times comfortably.
2. Do ten repetitions of the exercise at each station.
3. Begin with just one round or bout of this workout and work your way to three bouts of the workout at each station.

You will become stronger each week (or every other week if you train only three times a week) so you will have to increase the number of pounds you lift. That way, you will be getting stronger gradually. You only have to work on those stations that exercise parts of the body where you feel the need to increase your strength, such as the parts of the body infrequently used in your other activities.

You will find this piece of equipment and the free weights at most gyms or at high schools and universities. (Check YMCAs or YWCAs, too.)

Nautilus Equipment

Nautilus equipment (Fig. 2) not only is found in some high schools and universities, but in fitness centers by that name. This equipment essentially gives you the same opportunity for strength development as the Universal Gym, and it may be easier for you to locate, but by belonging to a Nautilus center, you also have the advantage of knowing when you can work out.

The equipment, like the less elaborate Universal Gym, gives you strength gain and muscular endurance. Also, if workouts are executed according to direction, the Nautilus equipment is said to improve flexibility because you do the exercises throughout the range of motion. (This can be done on the Universal Gym, too, but it isn't designed in quite the same way to enhance flexibility training.)

There is no cardiovascular development gained from weight training programs. Therefore, you would have to supplement weight training with a cardiovascular activity in order to get maximum fitness development. We suggest also that you supplement weight training with flexibility exercises for all parts of the body.

Here is one workout that you can do on the Nautilus equipment:

Leg extensions • two sets of fifteen

Leg curls • two sets of fifteen

Hip machine • two sets of ten for each leg

Double chest machine

    Fly and bench press • two sets of ten to twelve

Double shoulder

    Lateral raise • two sets of ten to twelve

    Seated press • two sets of ten to twelve

All other machines • two sets of ten each

Health spas and fitness centers are business ventures; keep this in mind. Many women truly enjoy such places because there is a kind of camaraderie in women exercising together. If this appeals to you, then by all means partake in it. Just remember that the information the health spas can give may be less than adequate and possibly incorrect.

Also, some of the equipment they claim will work wonders for your body won't do a darn thing but bruise you. (For example, the roller machine you sit on that is supposed to roll off the fat or the belt you put around your hips to "vibrate the fat off"— nonsense!) Good pieces of equipment such as the Universal Gym or the Nautilus would be far more beneficial.

Keep in mind that when you test yourself periodically on a piece of spa equipment, it is important to test yourself on the same piece of equipment that you have been training on. In other words, don't lift free weights and then go test yourself on the Nautilus equipment. They are two different pieces of equipment and will give you different results.

Be sure that if you put your hard-earned money into a health spa or fitness center that you get your money's worth from it. You should use the center at least twice a week and preferably more, so schedule your time so you can do this. It might help if you find out when the facility isn't crowded so that you will be less apt to be hindered in your workout.

Table 2
Activities Rated According to Physical Fitness Benefits
(Flexibility, Strength, Cardiovascular Endurance)

	Flexibility	Upper Body (Strength)	Lower Body (Strength)	Cardio-Vascular Endurance	RATING 1—Poor 2—Fair 3—Average 4—Good 5—Excellent
Walking			x		1
Slowly			x		1
Briskly			x	x	2
Running			x	x	3
Running Program*	x	x	x	x	5
Bicycling			x	x	3
Swimming (All basic strokes)	x	x	x	x	5
Kayaking		x			2
Canoeing		x			2
Sailing					
Small Boats	x	x	x		3
Large Boats					1
Rowing	x	x			2
Horseback Riding			x	x	3
Karate (Martial Arts)	x	x	x	x	5
Bowling		x	x		1
Ballet	x		x		4
Folk Dance			x	x	3
Square Dance			x	x	3
Modern Dance	x	x	x	x	5
Aerobic Dance	x	x	x	x	5
Gymnastics	x	x	x	x	5
Backpacking		x	x		2
Golf					
Walking		x	x		2
Cart		x			1
Snow Skiing					
Alpine	x		x	x	4
Nordic	x	x	x	x	5
Water Skiing		x	x		3
Mountain Climbing	x	x	x	x	5
Yoga	x				2
Weight Lifting		x	x		2
Tennis					
Singles	x	x	x	x	4
Doubles	x	x	x		3
Badminton	x	x	x	x	4
Racquetball	x	x	x	x	5
Field Hockey	x	x	x	x	4
Basketball	x	x	x	x	4
Soccer	x	x	x	x	5
Softball	x	x	x	x	3
Volleyball	x	x	x	x	4

* Running combined with upper body flexibility and strength exercises.

With a bird's-eye view of several different kinds of activities and the knowledge of the level of fitness you should expect to obtain, your job now is to find some activity you enjoy and to become involved in that activity (see Table 2). Check to see if your program might be lacking in one area of the fitness components and if other activities or exercises are needed as supplements. There are many ways to be physically active, to get reasonably fit, and to enjoy it too!

5

Diet and
Weight Control

A prime motivation for many women who enter into an exercise program is the desire to lose weight. It is also possible for some women to enter into an activity program with the hope of gaining weight, or simply of maintaining their weight.

However, it seems to be true that the largest number of women who wish to begin exercising are those who find themselves overweight and flabby.

Exercise alone is usually not sufficient to cause weight loss. *The best way to lose weight is to combine exercise with a proper nutritional program.* Women who begin to jog, play tennis, or enter into some other activity expect to see the pounds melt away and are extremely disappointed when this doesn't happen. On the other hand, some women begin to exercise and, at the same time, begin some type of extreme, totally unsuitable, dietary regime for weight loss. As a result, not only do they lose weight, but they find themselves totally fatigued, and even ill.

To lose weight (or for that matter to gain weight) takes a significant amount of time. Overnight weight reduction or weight increase is not practical, feasible, or sensible and, in fact, it can be downright dangerous! Many books written about these kinds of diets, even books written by doctors, have been condemned by the medical profession. Following such regimens could cause many complications in your health.

Not only has book publishing flourished as a result of the diet fads that exist today, but there are many individuals who prey on the gullible person who wants to lose weight and doesn't want to work to do it. This type of person goes to facilities to be shaken by machines, doused with water, exercised too vigorously, and "sauna-ized" for a long period of time, only to be left weaker and poorer. Others go to "diet farms" where they are put on strict diets. They lose weight while they are at the farm, but because it is a forced diet over a short period of time, they soon put the weight back on when they return home where no one is watching what they eat.

Among the more ridiculous books and articles that have been written are those concerning "cellulite." In these, the author tries to convince you that massage of this so-called cellulite breaks up the fat. This is utter nonsense. Fat is fat, and there is no such thing as cellulite. It is nothing different, just plain, ordinary fat.

One of the most dangerous diets that has been popular recently is the liquid protein diet. This type of diet regimen has to be controlled by very strict medical supervision, or the patient may become extremely ill. In fact, deaths have occurred from unsupervised use of liquid protein as a method of rapid weight reduction (when used as a person's sole dietary intake).

This type of dieting certainly is not recommended for the person who is attempting to achieve all-around physical fitness by exercise. To achieve fitness, you must combine your exercise with a normal (or modestly lower) caloric, well-balanced diet, defined as one that meets the standards set by the Committee on Recommended Dietary Allowances of the Food and Nutrition Board, National Research Council, National Academy of Sciences. We will discuss such a diet shortly.

Physiological Considerations

You will have to know a little bit about the physiology of your body to understand calories, energy production, and metabolism.

Energy produced in your body is measured in a unit called a *calorie*, scientifically defined as the amount of heat necessary to raise one gram of water one degree Celsius. When we talk about the number of calories burned by the body, we use a term that actually is a thousand times the basic unit of a calorie, a *kilogram calorie*. This kilogram calorie, then, is the technically correct unit used to measure the amount of energy that is stored in our body, but we will simply refer to it as a calorie.

The next question, then, is where does this energy that we are measuring with calories come from? When energy is produced in the body the process by which it occurs is known as *metabolism*. This process goes on in many places in our bodies and we fuel this energy with the food we eat.

There are three basic types of food, which we label protein, fat, and carbohydrate. Fat contains the largest amount of calories (nine per gram), while both protein and carbohydrate produce four calories.

You all know what fat is. It is found in most meats in its purest form, but it's also seen in many other foods, and it may be an additive in cooking and baking. Proteins are also found mainly in meats, but may be found in many vegetables. Carbohydrates are found in about all food substances that contain sugar and starch, and therefore would be found in most vegetables, all bread products, fruits, and even in some meat products, particularly those such as cereal-fortified hamburgers, hot dogs, and sausages.

After food is eaten and passed into the stomach, it is attacked by hydrochloric acid. Then it is digested in the small intestine by specific enzymes. These enzymes act as catalysts to speed the rate of the chemical reactions that change the food into simpler compounds. These compounds are then absorbed through the walls of the intestines and into the bloodstream. There are many different types of enzymes, and each one acts upon a specific type of food to break it down so that it can be absorbed.

It generally takes two to three hours for food to be absorbed by the intestinal tract and to then become available as energy for the body. Food materials that are not digested finally exit the body through the rectum. Waste products from the tissues that are in the blood are filtered out by the kidneys and leave the body as urine. Another waste product, carbon dioxide, is exhaled through the lungs.

Many of the food substances that have been broken down

and absorbed are stored in the form of a substance called glycogen in the liver. This stored substance can be mobilized when needed for physical activity or, in time of stress, released into the bloodstream. To do this, the body must have an adequate supply of oxygen, because it can function for only a very limited time on "anaerobic" energy (the energy available to the muscles in the absence of oxygen).

When energy is needed, the liver breaks down some of its stored glycogen and releases it into the bloodstream as glucose, which is carried by the blood to the muscles and other tissues. The hormone insulin is stimulated by this release of glucose, and this facilitates the entry of glucose into the tissue cells where it is needed for energy production. Oxygen is necessary for the glucose to be broken down into a chemical form of energy.

After it has been used up, a waste product called lactic acid accumulates in the tissues, particularly in the muscles. Lactic acid needs to be removed from the tissues by the bloodstream and disposed of by the body. This is why it is so necessary that we speed up our circulation and our respiration when we exercise.

At some time, you have probably experienced what is called a "stitch" in your side when you have been running for a long time or exercising rapidly. You have had to stop for a moment and catch your breath as the pain disappears. It is believed that stitches are caused by a lack of oxygen in the intercostal muscles (those between the ribs) or in the diaphragm, and you must pause momentarily while the oxygen is replaced.

You also may have experienced what is called "second wind." This occurs when you seem to be getting more and more fatigued and short of breath, and then, all of a sudden, you find yourself able to begin breathing normally again and to continue your activity without limitation. We believe this is because your body makes an adjustment in your energy requirements by restoring oxygen and glucose to your muscles while balancing the electrolytes (sodium, potassium, chloride, calcium, and so forth) in the tissues.

The body is a delicate machine that requires fuel to keep it running. It needs this fuel in balanced amounts, and it needs an equal supply of the catalyst enzymes, hormones, and so on to keep it going and to keep all the elements involved in balance. To do this requires a proper diet.

Proper Diet

Studies have shown that people who do not eat regularly, or who eat in an erratic fashion, are in poorer health than those who eat regular meals. People who eat breakfast almost every day have been found to have a higher energy level than people of the same age who do not eat breakfast. It also has been shown that people who don't eat between meals, or who only occasionally eat between meals, are healthier than those who regularly eat between meals. Irregular eating also results in overweight, further decreasing the overall health status.

The foremost rule in eating a proper diet is to eat regularly, usually three meals a day. There are people whose metabolisms work at a faster rate, thus requiring that they eat as many as four or five meals a day to maintain their weight. Generally, these people eat smaller quantities. There is nothing wrong with this, and sometimes it is even advisable for people who are trying to stay on a diet.

Calories

The amount of calories required in your diet will depend on a number of factors, including your height and age. For instance, when we are younger we require more calories than when we are older.

Our caloric requirements until we reach age twenty-one and cease growing are much higher than after we are physically matured and trying to maintain a fixed weight. When we become older, our ways become more sedentary and we therefore require fewer calories.

Thus, there is no fixed number of calories that we can state as a general rule. There are, however, *average* amounts of calories for various groups of people who are employed in various categories.

The average-sized woman who is a housewife generally will require 1,600 to 1,800 calories a day, depending on the size of her family and how much housework (laundry, running up and down stairs, cleaning, chasing the children) she does. An office secretary, sitting at a typewriter all day, will require only 1,625 calories a day, depending on her other activities.

The professional soldier in battle or undergoing rigorous training may require anywhere from 4,000 to 6,000 calories a day. The growing teenager who is fairly active would probably require around 3,000 to 3,500 calories a day.

Thus, some knowledge of the amount of calories we consume is very important. There are many calorie charts available on the market, usually in small paperback form, which give the caloric content of various portions of food. There are also little pocket guides that you can keep in your purse and refer to when you are eating out if you are trying to maintain a strict calorie count.

Balancing Your Diet

In addition to keeping in mind the number of calories you consume, you must remember to include in your diet a good balance of protein, fat, and carbohydrates. Determine the number of grams of protein, carbohydrates, and fat in your diet.

Protein: 20 percent of total calories for growing children and pregnant women, minimum of 0.5 grams/pound of desirable body weight for other adults (0.04 ounce = 1 gram).
Carbohydrate: from 50 to 70 percent of nonprotein calories.
Fat: from 30 to 50 percent of nonprotein calories.

There are recommended dietary allowances (called "RDA") for adults and children of more than four years of age, and these include, among other items, 45 or 65 grams (1.6 ounces) of protein each day. The Committee on Recommended Dietary Allowances also lists the daily allowance of nutrients required in addition to protein, such as vitamins and minerals (Table 3).

Protein, of course, is probably the most important basic food because it functions to build and repair all of the body tissues and is the major source of supplying energy. Good sources of protein are such things as meat, fish, poultry, eggs, milk, and cheese, and it is also found in dry peas, beans, peanuts, and enriched breads and cereals.

Carbohydrates are basically a high energy food substance, and for quick energy you would want to eat foods with a high concentration of these. Carbohydrates are found in all sweets,

Table 3
Recommended Dietary Allowance (RDA)
For Adults and Children More Than Four Years Old

Nutrients (required listing)	Amounts
Protein	45 or 65 grams**
Vitamin A	4,000 International Units
Vitamin C (ascorbic acid)	45 milligrams
Thiamine (vitamin B_1)	1.1 milligrams
Riboflavin (vitamin B_2)	1.2 milligrams
Niacin	12–16 milligrams
Calcium	800 milligrams
Iron	18 milligrams

**45 grams if protein quality is equal to or greater than milk protein; 65 grams if protein quality is less than milk protein.

Nutrients (optional listing)	Amounts
Vitamin D	400 International Units
Vitamin E	12 International Units
Vitamin B	2.0 milligrams
Folic acid[6] (folacin)	400 micrograms
Vitamin B_{12}	3.0 micrograms
Phosphorus	1.0 gram
Iodine	150 micrograms
Magnesium	300 milligrams
Zinc	15 milligrams
Copper	2 milligrams
Biotin	0.3 milligrams
Pantothenic acid	10 milligrams

sugar, starches, cereals, breads, rice, pasta, and potatoes.

The most concentrated source of food energy is fat, containing as we mentioned nine calories a gram as opposed to four for protein and carbohydrates. However, too much of a good thing can cause you to gain weight. Sources of fat include margarine, vegetable oils, butter, salad dressings, nuts, meat, and dairy fats such as cream cheese.

Many vitamins are essential to good health. The major ones include A, C, D, B1, B2, and niacin. Vitamin A is important for vision and is found in such things as eggs, liver, dark green and yellow vegetables, butter, margarine, milk, peaches, and cantaloupe.

Vitamin D is essential because it helps the body utilize calcium and phosphorus, which are important for our teeth and bones. Good sources of vitamin D include fortified milk, margarine, fish liver oils, and some vegetables such as carrots. It is also formed in the skin when exposed to sunlight (although, as we now know, too much sunlight can be dangerous).

Vitamin C, ascorbic acid, is very important, being necessary for healthy tissues of such areas as the gums, blood vessels, bones, and teeth. It also is known to promote healing. Vitamin C is found primarily in various citrus fruits, berries such as strawberries, cantaloupe, broccoli, cabbage, tomatoes, green peppers, and potatoes.

Thiamin or vitamin B1 is important for digestion and helps maintain a healthy nervous system. A good source for it is meat (especially pork and liver), enriched breads, cereals, dried peas, and beans.

Vitamin B2, riboflavin, is also important to keep the nervous system functioning properly, and also the eyes, skin, and mouth tissues. Good sources for it include meat (especially liver), milk, eggs, enriched breads, cereals, and green leafy vegetables.

Last among the vitamin group is niacin, another important aid for the nervous system, the skin, and the mouth. It is found in fish and certain meats (particularly liver), enriched bread, cereals, milk, and peanuts.

In addition to vitamins, we need certain minerals. Calcium is needed for healthy bones and teeth, nerves, muscles, and heart function. It is found particularly in milk products, but also in such fish as salmon and sardines, and in green leafy vegetables. Last, but not least, we need iron, which functions to help build red blood cells. Good sources for iron include meat (especially liver), egg yolks, oysters, green leafy vegetables, dried fruits, and enriched breads and cereals.

A proper diet of three regular meals a day should include, for breakfast, citrus fruit or fruit juice, cereal or an egg, and milk.

Luncheon for most people is the lightest meal, although it can also be the main meal. It may be varied and can include such popular foods as hamburgers or hot dogs, but it is better to include a variety of foods such as soups, salads, and other sandwiches. The main meal, dinner, usually should consist of a salad or some type of fruit or soup as an appetizer, followed by a green or yellow vegetable, a white vegetable such as potatoes, turnips or parsnips, and lean meat, fish, or fowl. Dinner may then be followed by a dessert, the amount or type depending upon the content of the main meal. With a heavier meal that includes potatoes or beans, for example, one might want to eat a light dessert such as jello. With a lighter dinner of perhaps two leafy green vegetables and lean meat, one might then allow a heavier dessert such as cake or pie.

Additives

A few comments should be made about food ingredients and additives. Additives generally are approved for use by the Food and Drug Administration and are permitted in certain products that are carefully controlled by the United States Department of Agriculture. Additives may be defined as substances used to increase flavor, improve color or texture, or improve the keeping qualities of food. They do not, as a general rule, add to the nutrient value of the food unless the additives are vitamins or minerals. Of course, we might say that spices, which are commonly used in all of our foods, are additives, and that as we add salt to our food we are using an additive. However, we are more concerned about those types of *chemical* products that are added to foods, such as sodium nitrites or dye additives used for coloring. Sugar and spices are more commonly referred to as ingredients.

Recently some of these food additives, such as nitrites, have been suggested to be carcinogenic. However, nitrites are important in preserving meats such as weiners and ham, preventing the growth of botulin. If evidence continues to show a deleterious effect, these additives may be removed, particularly from prepared meats.

When buying food, read the label and see what the product contains. You should know that, in accordance with the United

States Department of Agriculture regulations, ingredients must be listed in descending order of amount used by weight. Therefore, if the meat product itself is listed far down on the list, then there probably are more additives than meat in the weiner.

Determining Weight and Caloric Needs

If you wish to reduce your weight, not only must you reduce the number of calories you eat, but you must reduce them below the maintenance number of calories needed to keep your current weight.

First, determine your "ideal" weight for your height. If you have a medium build, allow 100 pounds for your first five feet of height and then add five pounds for each additional inch. If you have a small build, subtract 10 percent of the total number of pounds. If you have a large build, add 10 percent of the total number of pounds.

Now we will show you a relatively easy method for determining your caloric needs:

1. Basal calories equals desirable body weight (lb.) x 10   =_____

2. Add activity calories
   a. Sedentary equals desirable body weight (lb.) x 3   =+_____
   b. Moderate equals desirable body weight (lb.) x 5   =+_____
   c. Strenuous equals desirable body weight (lb.) x 10   =+_____

3. Add calories for indicated weight gain, growth (pregnant women), or lactation.   =+_____

4. Subtract calories for indicated weight loss.   =-_____

For example, say you have been eating 2,000 calories a day and gaining weight. If your desired weight is 125 pounds and your activity level is sedentary, you should be consuming only 1,625 calories. If you only drop your dietary intake to 1,625 calories, however, you simply will maintain the weight you now have. You will have *stopped* gaining weight, but you won't *lose* the extra weight previously gained even though your caloric intake has been reduced.

There are many publications available which will tell you what to eat to lose weight *sensibly. You should lose no more than two to three pounds a week.* You can calculate how much you need to reduce your caloric intake to gain this desired goal by consulting the following chart:

1. Basal calories: desired body weight x 10   =_____

2. Activity calories

     a. Sedentary: desirable body weight x 3   =+_____

     b. Moderate: desirable body weight x 5   =+_____

     c. Strenuous: desirable body weight x 10   =+_____

3. Growth calories

     a. Pregnancy: add 300 calories a day to gain 23 lbs. in 9 months (add calcium to provide 1.5 grams a day and supplement vitamins if needed)   =+_____

     b. Lactation: add 500 calories a day   =+_____

     c. To gain 1 lb. per week, add 500 calories a day   =+_____

4. To lose 1 lb. a week, subtract 500 calories a day   =-_____

                  Total Calories Needed   =_____

For example, if you now weigh 140 pounds and the caloric intake required to maintain that weight is 1,690 calories, but you wish to lose one pound a week, then you must drop your caloric intake to 1,190 calories. If you wish to lose at a faster rate, at least initially, you can drop that amount below 1,000 calories a day. However, if you become weak and dizzy, or you can't carry out assigned tasks, this is a sign of too much caloric reduction. It makes sense to lose weight at a slower rate and to maintain your general health than to attempt a crash diet and become sick in the process.

This is one of the reasons many people give up reducing diets. They attempt a crash diet to lose weight rapidly and become so irritable, so unhappy, and so discomforted by it that in a very short time they give it up. In addition, if they do persist with the diet despite the discomfort and they do reach the weight that they want, most people then promptly go back to eating what they were eating before and end up gaining all the weight back again.

If you take the slower route your body will adjust gradually and your desire to eat will be decreased. As a result, when you do get down to the weight you wish to retain, you will find it much easier to eat only that number of calories needed to maintain this desired weight.

There have been many crash diets introduced such as the high-protein-low-carbohydrate diet in which you only eat meat, drink water and take vitamins. This type of diet, however, produces "ketosis," the production of acetone wastes in the body, and individuals who continue this diet for any length of time can become very ill. The liquid protein diets, if undertaken without supervision, also can result in severe metabolic imbalance resulting from an overabundance of protein.

One of the biggest factors in any attempt to reduce your weight is overcoming psychological barriers. Why do most of us overeat? Is it just that we like food so much that we want to stuff ourselves? No, this usually is not the case. Most of us overeat because we are in some way fighting frustration, disappointment, job dissatisfaction, or family problems.

Some people eat when they get nervous, some people eat when they are happy. There is no one factor, psychologically,

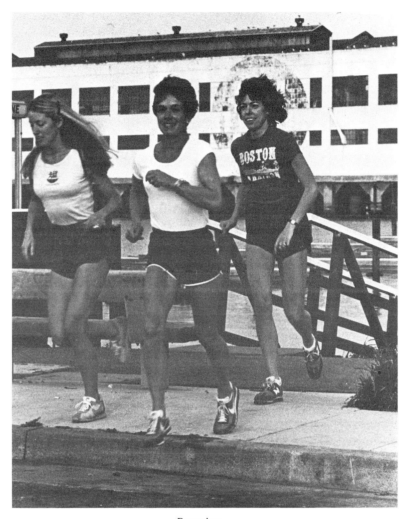

Running

that causes us to do it, but it's there and when we can't control these factors we continue to eat.

This theory of psychological causes for overeating has resulted in the success of programs that emphasize a group-therapy approach. Finding oneself among other people with similar problems who are banding together and giving each other help aids persistence in adhering to a diet that sometimes cannot be done alone. This appears to be the most successful approach toward a dietary program.

If you are not the joining type, or do not like the idea of belonging to an organization specifically to help yourself lose weight, there are many other kinds of groups (YMCAs, YWCAs, churches, schools, and so on) to help you.

You sometimes can do it just by banding together with two or three of your neighbors. Here you can put up such incentives as little contests to see who can lose their required weight each week. For example, if you don't lose the two pounds a week that you have set as a goal, you have to put some money in the kitty. Accumulate this money until the time when you've all reached your desired weights, and then you can celebrate.

Any such psychological maneuver will make it easier for you to lose weight. The desire to eat is so intense for some women that only by absolute isolation from everyone, such as at a health farm where all intake is carefully monitored, can they reduce weight. For a few women, it would take being stranded on a desert island.

If you do not wish simply to reduce your caloric intake to lose weight, you can bring about weight reduction by a minimum reduction in your caloric intake, but a marked increase in your physical activity. Combining physical activity with reduction of caloric intake is more sensible and easier on your body as well.

The number of calories consumed per hour by the average person has been calculated for various sports and activities. For example, we know that rope skipping consumes about 300 calories an hour if done leisurely and about 800 calories an hour if done vigorously. Jogging at a very slow pace of twelve minutes per mile (5 m.p.h.) consumes about 450 to 600 calories an hour. Running at a fast pace of six minutes per mile (10 m.p.h.), on the other hand, consumes 900 to 1285 calories.

Other activities, such as handball, consume 600 calories an hour. Pitching softball consumes 300 calories an hour, horseback riding at a trot consumes about 360 calories an hour, ice hockey 600 calories an hour, and riding a motorcycle about 200 calories an hour.

If you don't want to engage in sports, there are activities around the house that you can do to increase your caloric consumption. Raking leaves, for example, burns up 360 calories an hour, gardening with much lifting, stooping, and digging uses up 360 calories an hour, and scrubbing the floor burns about 250 calories an hour.

Various conditioning exercises, already mentioned in previous chapters, are another way to use up calories. Check in nutrition or diet and weight control books for charts on energy expenditure for various activities.

Physical fitness is very dependent upon the type of diet you eat, the activities you perform, and the way you watch your calorie consumption. To maintain a physically fit body you must eat a properly balanced diet, exercise at least moderately, and follow other simple rules of good health that include: proper sleep (generally seven to eight hours a night), a minimum consumption of alcoholic beverages (which, incidentally, have a high caloric value), and avoidance of smoking (with its well-known dangers). It is also wise to take a short rest during the day, when indicated, after severe exercise or exertion. By following these simple rules, you can maintain physical fitness and be the person you want to be.

6

Injuries

When Title IX was developed in 1973 to provide equal opportunities for women to engage in sports at grade school, high school, and college levels, it also stirred nationwide interest in all types of sports activity for women who were no longer in school or college. The number of women participating in sports has increased dramatically.

For example, it is estimated that of the 25 million people in the United States who are jogging, half are women. There has also been a dramatic increase in women's participation in other sports, particularly tennis, bicycling, racquetball, golf, and swimming, and in team sports such as volleyball, basketball, and ice hockey.

Initially it was predicted, and to some extent it was true, that accompanying this increase in women's participation would be an increase in the numbers of injuries among the women participants. Athletic trainer Joan Gillette and co-author Christine Haycock conducted a survey of the types and number of injuries occurring at the collegiate level in sports when the Title IX activity first began (1973 to 1975). During this period, the number of women engaging in sports at the collegiate level doubled, so it was anticipated that the survey would show a proportionately larger number of injuries. When we did our survey we were also interested in what physical education people thought was the reason for the increased number of injuries among women.

The results of this survey were published in "Injuries to Women Athletes—Myth vs. Reality," a paper that appeared in the *Journal of the American Medical Association* in 1976. First, the results showed that the types of injuries women were sustaining were basically no different than those that male athletes had been sustaining for many years. Secondly, most of these injuries were related to the knees and ankles. It was discovered, however, that women were sustaining less severe injuries since they were not engaging in violent contact sports. For example, women did not suffer as many fractures or head injuries as the men.

The study also showed that injuries related entirely to anatomical differences between males and females were minor. For example, women sustained minor injuries to the vagina by water skiing, and in certain other sports there were minor injuries to the breasts. The primary injuries sustained by women were injuries to the knees resulting in chondromalacia (inflammation of the cartilage), an injury known as "shin splints," and another injury known as "stress fractures."

Shin splints are pains in the anterior part of the lower legs. Although there have been many theories as to its cause, in general we feel that it is the result of fatigue. It is probably associated with poor conditioning, as are many of the other injuries that initially were being sustained by women athletes.

Other injuries to the knee were thought to be anatomical in nature inasmuch as the female's pelvis is wider than the male's. The wider pelvis causes the woman's legs to hang down in a knock-kneed fashion from the hips to the knees. This increased angle results in more stress on the knee and consequently, dislocation of the kneecap is more likely.

Stress fractures are small fractures sustained from repetitive loading on the bone or bones, frequently occurring in the ankle. It is thought that stress fractures are often caused by poor conditioning, or poor pretraining prior to strenuous exercise.

Let us explain what is meant by preconditioning or pretraining. Over the years on boys' teams, where coaches and trainers were available, a player never went out on the playing field and immediately began to play football. He was always conditioned by exercises prior to actually going out and playing the game. This conditioning or warming up, with basic types of exercises, prepares the player by increasing his muscle performance ability before he actually goes onto the field. Many players perform a set of routine exercises for the entire summer at home before they begin game practice in the fall. Additional group exercises are added when fall practice begins. Before each game, they go through an exercise routine to "condition" for the game.

Many women, even at the collegiate and high school levels, never received this type of training, and therefore, have not formed the habit of preseason conditioning, or even a simple warm-up before engaging in exercise. Until recently, those of us who played in sports such as softball and basketball were never taught the value of a good exercise program before participation in the game. We would come out the first day of the season and begin to play. When you do this, you can expect to suffer more strains, sprains, and muscle pulls than if you condition yourself prior to starting.

As a result of this lack of conditioning, women particularly at the college level (where the greatest entry into sporting activities occurred) were in poor physical condition in many cases, and sustained a much larger number of injuries than they should have. Since conditioning programs have now been developed for women as well as men, the injury rate is dropping. Subsequent studies have now documented this decreasing number of injuries.

There have now been several studies done on the women cadets at the military academies in the United States. These women have been put through various stressful training programs and still are coming out in great shape. Initially, many women who entered these academy programs were unable to maintain the proficiency necessary to continue at the institutions, so at first, quite a number of women did drop out. However, those remaining continued to improve physically. Although in most instances they were not expected to reach the same level as their male colleagues, they improved their performances remarkably in the few years that these programs have been in existence. It is anticipated that even more improvement will be shown as time progresses.

Importance of Conditioning

Certainly if you plan to enter a new sport, you should condition for it. For instance, if you decide to learn to ski, it is extremely important that you get a good instructor, or at least buy a good book on skiing and read about conditioning. Skiing can be a very dangerous sport, and many of the fractures that men and women sustain occur because of poor physical conditioning beforehand.

The same thing applies to any other new sport, whether it be tennis, swimming, golf, or whatever you plan to do. Find out what exercises will best put you in condition to play that sport, and make them a religious part of your preplay routine. If you do, you will not only be more proficient at the sport, but you will be able to enjoy it without as much risk of injury. This conditioning can go on all year long, not just during the season that you are playing in a particular sport.

No matter how well conditioned you are, however, some injuries are going to occur in any sport played vigorously. When injuries do occur, there are certain simple, basic treatments that should be followed.

Simple muscle pulls or strains. A muscle pull or strain usually means that there are a few fibers torn in the muscle. When this happens, there is a little bleeding into the muscle and swelling. As a result, there will be pain in the muscle and you will have difficulty moving the body part that the muscle controls.

Sprains. A more serious injury is a sprain, examples of which would be turning your ankle or twisting your wrist. It is not just an injury within a muscle bundle, but is an actual stretch or tear of the tendons, a pulling on nerves and blood vessels, and can be associated with fractures. Of course, if a fracture occurs you must seek medical advice immediately, and if it's a severe sprain with much pain and swelling, you certainly should be seen by a physician. However, it is not necessary that a physician see every slight sprain, particularly when there obviously is no significant amount of swelling, dislocation, or severe pain in the injured joint.

A simple sprain results in a small amount of swelling and a little tenderness, but you are still able to use the affected part.

The best first-aid method for such an injury is to pack the injured area in ice *immediately.* Prompt application of ice reduces the amount of swelling, and hence minimizes the pain and discomfort you have the following day.

Commercial cold packs are available in which you simply squeeze a bag to release a chemical that produces cold. Then you merely apply the plastic bag to the injured part. However, you can simply use crushed ice or, if you don't have crushed ice, crack up ice cubes, put them into a double plastic bag, and then apply the bag to the injury with a thin sheet or thin towel between the bag and skin. Placing the cloth between the bags and the skin prevents the possibility of the skin becoming blistered or actually burned from the ice.

The ice should be kept on the injured area for a minimum of twenty to thirty minutes. In addition the limb should be elevated, ideally to the level of the heart. However, in case of an ankle, elevating it at least to the level of the pelvis by sitting with your feet up on a stool or ottoman will suffice. This enhances the return of waste products from the injured area and allows additional circulation, which will help reduce swelling and discomfort.

If the limb is left hanging down, edema (excessive accumulation of fluid) will result, impeding circulation and removal of waste products. Thus it is very important that the injured area be elevated. If a wrist or arm is injured, it can be placed in a sling and kept above the heart. Following (or with) the application of ice, the injured area can be wrapped firmly with an elastic bandage and the elevation continued.

When you go to bed, continue to maintain the elevation of the injured part by placing it on pillows. If the strain is severe and skin discoloration is present the following morning, it might then be advisable to report to an emergency room for an X-ray of the injured part just to be certain that there is no fracture.

If the sprain is moderately severe, but there is no fracture, you may find it advisable to remain at home and rest the injured part for a day or two. During this time, however, motion should be encouraged without bearing weight on the area. After this, the use of an ankle or wrist support may make it easier for you to walk about or use your arm for a week or so. However, you should expect to be able to move about within that time.

Muscle pulls and strains can take up to six or eight weeks to heal, depending upon the severity and type of initial injury. If you have any doubt about the seriousness of the injury, you should consult your physician. Aspirin, or buffered aspirin, can be used for pain, or, if you cannot take aspirin, you can use a substitute product. Aspirin is a good antiinflammatory agent readily available in the home, and it is preferable to aspirin substitutes if you are able to take it.

Scrapes and scratches. In any type of sport you can expect to sustain some minimal scrapes and scratches. Those injuries resulting in deep lacerations will require the services of a physician to clean and suture them. Small scrapes and scratches can be treated by the athlete herself.

These injuries should be cleansed immediately using a mild soap and water or such products as pHisohex or Betadine, if available. All dirt and foreign matter such as gravel or dirt should be removed carefully from the would. After cleansing the wound thoroughly and irrigating it well with water, an antiseptic agent such as iodine or Merthiolate may then be applied. Finally, the area should be covered with a sterile bandage.

Scrapes and scratches must be kept clean, and if you are going to continue to play, it is important that the area be kept covered and then recleaned after playing. It is best to keep scratches and scrapes of the skin clean and exposed to the air when you are at home to enable the area to dry out and provide a normal scab cover. Keeping the area covered at all times with a bandage excludes oxygen from the area and retards healing. If, however, you must go out, you should then cover it.

All areas of scrapes and scratches should be watched for any increasing redness or swelling, which might indicate the onset of infection. If such symptoms appear, you should consult your physician immediately.

It is also important to have had a booster shot against tetanus within the last five years before engaging in any sport in which you may suffer an injury. Tetanus boosters are relatively innocuous and produce very little in the way of symptoms.

Weather and Health

Something else that you must take into consideration is the weather. If you are going to be exercising in an area that is either very cold or very hot, it is sometimes necessary to acclimatize yourself (adjust to the environment) before beginning. Sometimes it is necessary to spend a few days at a location before beginning a sports activity to adjust to such things as altitude, humidity, or temperature. This might be the case, for example, if you were going to Denver to play tennis. There the altitude is such that the oxygen content of the air is slightly reduced over that at lower levels, and possible shortness of breath could cause you some difficulty in playing a match.

The weather also determines appropriate attire. For example, if you are going skiing it is very important that you wear proper clothing. It must be a kind that will enable your body to maintain its temperature and yet avoid unnecessary loss of heat through sweating. It is also a good idea to go outside and stay outside for half an hour or so before you begin skiing so that you adjust properly to the temperature.

In cold weather, layered types of clothing are good because as you begin to warm up, you are able to remove a layer or two of clothing and then put it back on if you become colder, or when you finish exercising. In a way, cold temperatures are easier to adapt to than heat because you have the ability to add or remove clothing.

In the heat, there is a limit to how much clothing you can remove since normally we cannot play in the nude. When no further removal of clothing is possible and you are very hot, it might be best to sit down in the shade with a cold drink for a while. Of course, you can't very well do this if you are in the middle of athletic competition, so learning to adapt to the heat is very important.

People respond differently to heat. Your body build may have an affect on how well you can dissipate heat. Someone who is short and stocky, or a little on the chubby side, will tend to retain more heat than someone who is thin. A high percentage of body fat sometimes acts as an insulator and makes it hard for a person to tolerate heat.

As in cold weather, the type of clothing you wear in the heat is important. Synthetic materials, such as nylon, tend to retain heat and do not absorb sweat, whereas cotton materials not only absorb sweat, but radiate heat better because cotton is more porous. This allows evaporation, which in turn increases cooling.

You should never limit the amount of liquids you drink when you are sweating. There have been many old wives' tales that if you drink too much water when it's hot, you'll get stomach cramps. As a result, athletes in the past have limited their intake of fluids, causing many to pass out in the heat and some even to die.

Acclimatizing to a new environment takes four to ten days. If you simply exercise sensibly, wear proper clothing, and drink plenty of liquids to make up for the fluid you lose in sweating, you should stay out of trouble.

Injuries in Particular Sports

There are types of injuries that are particularly identified with certain sports. Jogging, for example, which recently has become so popular, has resulted in problems associated with the feet. The wearing of improperly fitted shoes can result in blisters, calluses, and ankle sprains that can be very disabling to the jogger.

The best way to treat these types of injuries is to prevent them from happening in the first place. Wear properly fitted shoes. In addition, if you have any inherent difficulty with your feet, such as poor arches, bunions, or calluses, it would be best to consult a podiatrist familiar with athletes and about proper treatment rather than attempting to treat problems yourself.

However, if what you have is a very mild flattening of the longitudinal arch (the main arch of the foot), simply wearing a device such as a Scholl's arch support in your running shoe may be all that you need. If you already have been wearing arch supports in your everyday shoes, you might want to have them in your running shoes as well. If, after your shoes are properly broken in, you do get blisters or calluses, you must consider different shoes and treat these problems correctly.

Blisters should not be opened, because opening them may result in infection. It is best to simply pad the area and let the blister dry out by itself. (This is different from the type of treatment for burn blisters, in which your physician may elect to open them.) If the blister is already open because it has been rubbed by the shoe, then it is very important that it be thoroughly cleansed. The best way to do this is to soak your foot for ten minutes in a soapy solution and then gently and thoroughly scrub the area. Allow the area to dry, or dry it with a sterile pad and then paint it with iodine or Merthiolate and apply a sterile dressing. The area should be inspected daily for any swelling or redness with streaks going up the leg that might indicate infection. If this occurs, you should consult your physician immediately.

Two very common complaints associated with sports involving throwing a ball or using a racquet are "tennis elbow" and "racquetball wrist." There are many factors associated with the production of these injuries, but frequently they are atributed to poor playing habits. An improper backhand stroke, for example, is a common cause of tennis elbow, and an improper forehand stroke in racquetball can result in racquetball wrist. These injuries are an inflammation of the tendons, referred to as tendinitis. While there are methods of treatment such as warm water soaks, aspirin, and the use of such a device as a tennis elbow guard (which is applied to the muscles of the forearm), rest is usually required to allow healing of the injury.

If you develop tendinitis you may very well do so because you are overusing or misusing the musculoskeletal system of your elbow, wrist, or knee, as the case may be. This type of injury frequently occurs with beginning athletes and can be avoided if the player has proper instruction and uses proper equipment.

Tendinitis can be very painful and may, indeed, prevent you from being able to play until the pain subsides. Generally, tendinitis will subside, but it takes a number of weeks and if it becomes worse, you should see an orthopedic specialist to have the injury treated. In any event, some modification of your exercise routine is going to have to be made. In general, it means cutting down the activities that would involve using the affected part. Persistance in playing when you have tendinitis will result in aggravation of the injury, so you must give the part a chance to heal. There are exercise routines that can be used to

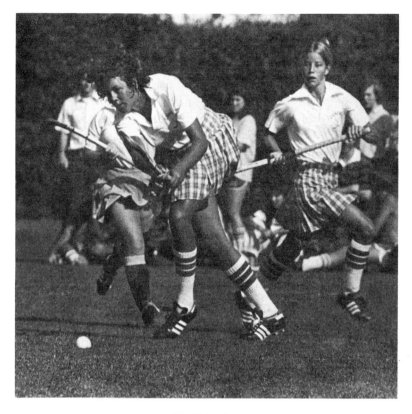

Field hockey

strengthen the affected areas gradually and permit you to use them again, but for this you need specialized help from a physiotherapist.

Playing softball can result in injuries to the shoulder from throwing. The woman who goes out on the softball field and begins to throw hard without warming her arm up (by throwing very gently at first) will certainly find herself with a pulled muscle, pinched nerve, or bursitis in her shoulder.

Field hockey players are subject to injuries to their shins from sticks and flying hockey balls. However, there seems to be a great tendency for women to feel that the wearing of shin guards is a "sissy" thing to do, and thus many refrain. This is, of course, very foolish because eventually, when they have been struck enough times on the shins so that they are bruised and bleeding, they will then *have* to wear the guards. And the guards themselves can rub and irritate the area. Prevention is again the key to avoiding such injuries.

Sources of injury from gym-related activites can be unsuitable floors, poorly devised training programs, improper gymnastic equipment, or unsupervised activities using gym equipment. Injuries to the hips and groin area occurring from slips and falls on gymnastic equipment can be very painful and can even cause hematomas (blood clots). The beginner in gymnastics should wear padding on vulnerable areas because it is not sufficient that the equipment itself be padded (although certainly it should be). Treatment for such injuries usually consists of soaking in a warm tub of water. However, more specialized treatment, such as physiotherapy, may be needed.

The older woman who is entering into an exercise or activity program, who previously has done little in the way of exercise, should be particularly careful. While she does not have to worry as much about her cardiovascular status as does an older man, such factors as arthritis, osteoporosis (thinning of the bones), and poorly conditioned muscles may cause her more injuries than her younger counterparts. Her entry into any new sport should be very slow and gradual to avoid problems.

In all cases we must aim at preventing the injury *before* it occurs. The use of proper equipment, proper clothing, and proper conditioning before exercise is the key to remaining uninjured. If you do suffer an injury, you can use common sense and first-aid treatment. However, if the injury is severe, or if it does not respond to home care, early treatment by a physician should be sought to prevent permanent damage. By obeying these rules you should be able to enjoy your participation in sports without any danger to your well-being.

7

Special Considerations of Active Women

One of the major concerns that women have always had in regard to physical activity is the effect that it might have on their menstrual periods and, at some future date, on pregnancy. We think exercise is good for both menstruation and pregnancy.

Menstruation is a complex process that involves the entire body and in particular the endocrine glands, uterus, ovaries, and vagina.

Your menstrual cycle is divided into three general phases termed premenstrual, menstrual, and intramenstrual. The average menstrual cycle extends more than 28 days, but of course this length of time varies among women, ranging anywhere from twenty-one to thirty-five days.

Problems of Menstruation

The premenstrual phase is usually the five days preceeding the actual menstrual flow, and it is the time during which much discomfort can occur from the retention of fluid by the body and the resultant tissue engorgement. Cramps may occur in the premenstrual phase and extend into the menstrual period, or they may begin only with the actual onset of the flow.

While the length of the menstrual period itself is usually three to five days, some women have periods that last only two or as many as seven days, lengths still considered normal.

During this flow a woman loses only one-and-a-half to five ounces of blood under normal circumstances. This small loss of blood is of absolutely no importance, and it generally is replaced by the formation of new blood cells in the bone marrow very quickly, so that anemia does not result.

However, women who have a very heavy flow of blood for longer than seven days may lose enough blood to become anemic, and such abnormal bleeding requires investigation by a physician. It may be an indication that there is an ovarian problem, or some type of growth in the uterus.

Some women do tend to run a lower red-blood count than average. If such women are indulging in athletic endeavors, it would be advantageous for them to take some type of an iron and vitamin supplement, because many anemias are the result of an iron-deficient dietary intake. Dr. Joan Ullyot of California has pointed this out in some excellent studies. She fed iron to her runners and was able to increase their performance, especially in long-distance running.

Certainly every woman should be checked to make sure she is not anemic when she is about to begin an exercise program. In general, however, anemia is not related to the menstrual flow unless there is some problem existent.

The onset of the menstrual period in girls in most areas of the world comes between the ages of twelve and fourteen, but it could range from nine to sixteen years. Recently, there have been studies indicating that this onset may be delayed until later in young girls training strenuously for competitive athletics. It has also been shown that the period will begin once the stressful training is discontinued.

This phenomenon not only occurs with the young athlete just beginning to menstruate, but it may also occur with older female athletes in very stressful training prior to important competition. This has been seen particularly in the sport of track and field. Exercise physiologists speculate that this is related to the percent of body fat a woman has. When the amount of fat is reduced below a certain undefined level, menstruation ceases.

Probably the most common female complaint however, is painful periods, or dysmenorrhea. Lower abdominal pains, cramps, and backaches accompanied at times by headaches, leg aches, breast fullness or tenderness, and nausea generally characterize this problem. While it most commonly occurs just at the beginning of the menstrual flow, it can occur even earlier and can last through the flow (although generally it stops when the flow is well established).

The amount of dysmenorrhea experienced is difficult to determine because of varying subjective factors and differences in pain tolerance among women. Gynecologists and others have estimated that 70 to 80 percent of the cases of painful menstruation can be attributed to faulty living habits, such as lack of exercise, poor posture, fatigue, irritability, and tension resulting from daily activities.

Effects of Menstruation on Exercise

There have been many studies done on the effects of menstruation on exercise. These have included measuring several aspects of physical performance, such as muscular strength and endurance, power of the legs, balance, steadiness, and distance running. The result of this testing has been inconclusive, however, and no fixed effect has been demonstrated. A well-motivated female athlete does not generally seem to allow her performance to be affected by her menstrual period.

There is no current evidence to suggest that participation in physical activity itself causes any significant change in the menstrual cycle, either favorably or unfavorably, for the majority of women. However, it can be said, and studies at the service academies have recently shown, that dysmenorrhea appears to be less common among healthy female athletes and physical education students than among those who are physically inactive. However, because of the pain tolerance factors that govern the reporting of the severity of symptoms, it is difficult to make an definitive statements.

The studies conducted at the service academies have shown that those women who engaged in strenuous physical activity during two years at the academy reported greatly reduced dysmenorrhea compared with what they experienced prior to their entrance into the academies. Therefore, we might conclude that this improvement was related to their improved physical condition.

Another aspect often discussed is whether or not there should be a restriction on physical activity or sports participation during any phase of the menstrual period. For the large majority of women, there is no such restriction. There has been no demonstrated harm from such activity during a normal menstruation. For example, professional women athletes need not stop their performances because they have a menstrual period. For that reason, there is no indication that any other woman should have to cease activity during her period.

The old wives' tales that have existed about not washing your hair, not swimming, not touching plants, and so forth during menstruation have absolutely no factual basis. Going back as far as the early 1920s, exercise has been recommended during the menstrual period to relieve discomfort. In general, these exercises involve systematic twisting and bending of the trunk and abdominal muscles, and include positions that strengthen the abdominal wall. These would include bent-knee sit-ups, trunk-twist exercises, and trunk-bending exercises.

Although we cannot guarantee that physical activity will do away with any painful periods that you may have, the odds are that it will help. We entertain no hesitation in recommending it for all women.

Pregnancy

Many outstanding women athletes who have had pregnancies and deliveries have been studied by investigators both in the United States and abroad. In general, these studies have indicated that these top athletes have a definite advantage over nonathletes in several factors related to pregnancy. These women have had shorter labors, less backache during pregnancy, fewer peritoneal tears during delivery, fewer incidences of cesarean section and forceps deliveries, and fewer manual removals of the afterbirth. In fact, it has been said that even among all of these women, the upper limits of what was considered a normal number of such incidents was never approached.

For that matter, a number of women marathon runners have continued to run until just prior to delivery. Several of these women were running as much as five miles a day right up to the day before delivery. In all of these instances, these women have reported minimal discomfort during labor, a fast labor, and no backache afterward.

Appropriate exercise during pregnancy has been advocated for many years, and we consider it a desirable thing. Such exercises, for example, have been stressed as a part of natural childbirth. A gradual physical conditioning program followed on an individually prescribed basis during a six-month to ten-month period, has been known to result in a steady reduction of pregnancy discomforts. From this we have seen that an exercise program can promote a normal delivery.

Another thing many women worry about is the possibility of injury to themselves or their developing babies if they indulge in physical activity during pregnancy. Studies carried out on exercise during pregnancy indicate that the child is protected in the uterus in such a way that the tough skin, muscles, tissues of the abdominal wall, and the thick uterine muscle lined by a membrane filled with embryonic fluid absorb the physical trauma encountered in the normal routine of the mother, and protect the growing fetus during physical activity.

Normal physical activity does not predispose the mother to miscarriage or injury. Obviously, a woman who is pregnant would not want to engage in a contact sport in which she might sustain a direct blow to the uterus. This would be foolish.

The type of exercise that is permitted or indicated during pregnancy is one that each woman must decide in consultation with her physician. A trained athlete might wish to sustain a higher level of activity than the housewife who is simply engaged in an exercise program. On the other hand, there is no necessity for a woman to worry about continuing physical activity, especially something like jogging, during her pregnancy.

Birth-Control Pills

While there is no major objection to active women using birth-control pills, they should be aware of the side effects that may occur, in particular the possibility of developing blood clots in the veins. Women on the birth-control pill may also suffer such adverse effects as headaches and nausea, especially when first beginning its use. Therefore, it would be inadvisable for an active woman to attempt to use the pill merely as a means to postpone her menstrual period (as some female athletes do before competition), especially if she has not been on the pill before.

Varicose Veins

Because of the increased incidence of blood clots in women on the pill, it has always been considered inadvisable for women who have varicose veins. In addition to this, women with varicose veins should also use some precautions when engaging in physical activity. It is advisable for such women to have their varicose veins attended to surgically, or to wear elastic supportive stockings during activity, because women who have large varicose veins and receive a blow to the leg could sustain a severe hemorrhage into the tissues. (This occurs because these veins are more easily ruptured than normal veins.) Fortunately, varicose veins are seldom a problem with young women actively participating in sports or physical activity.

Menopause

There are no known contraindications to the continuation of all sporting activities during menopause. In fact, quite the contrary is true, because engaging in sports during menopause can be particularly valuable.

Menopause, which usually occurs anywhere from age 45 upward, may be manifested by physical symptoms such as flushing and sweating, which frequently occurs during the night. Occasionally there are other physical symptoms, which include headache, insomnia, and episodes of dizziness. These symptoms can be controlled by the patient's physician either with the use of estrogen, or with other drugs. This matter should be resolved on an individual basis between the woman and her physician.

However, it is not the physical symptoms that represent the real problem. The major difficulties are the psychological ones that some women face as their menstrual period disappears. They feel they are now beyond the child bearing age and are facing the later years of their lives. For some women, this is a particularly depressing time and it may result in a psychosis known as "involutional melancholia." This can be a very severe form of illness requiring hospitalization for psychiatric care.

Most women, however, exhibit milder forms of this depression as manifested by anxiety, feelings of loneliness, and a sense of loss of well-being. A very negative effect upon all of their activites may occur. They become sluggish, tend to overeat, put on weight, and treat themselves as though they were really sick.

A healthy approach to this would be an increase in physical activity for a woman who has not been exercising. We have mentioned before the psychological importance of sports as a tension reliever, and this can be particularly valuable for the woman who is going through menopause.

By participating in a sport she can convince herself that she is not ready to put one foot in the grave just because this event has occurred, and that she has many good productive years of life ahead of her. By getting herself in good physical condition and keeping herself that way with exercise, she will be putting off the effects of aging that follow in the later years.

We mentioned the necessity of having the physical manifestations of the menopause controlled by medication administered by your physician and, of course, this involves having a complete physical examination. For those women who have not had hysterectomies, it must include a Pap smear.

Every woman should have a Pap smear at least once a year, and through the menopausal years it is advocated that a Pap smear be done twice a year, particularly if the woman is placed on estrogen during this time. An endometrial biopsy (the removing of a small piece of the lining of the uterus) is also recommended at least once a year.

Just doing a Pap smear, however, is not enough. A complete pelvic examination should be done, including bimanual and rectal examinations. (Women are not as prone to rectal cancer as men, so a yearly proctoscopic examination of the female is not indicated. However, should she have any symptoms such as changes in bowel habits, it certainly should be done.)

In addition to the Pap smear, women in this age group should have an EKG (electrocardiogram) done. This should then be repeated at suitable intervals by her family physician depending upon the findings on the initial EKG. If it is normal it may only be necessary to repeat it with the appearance of any symptoms of cardiac problems, or perhaps at five-year intervals. This is also true for chest X-rays unless the patient is, or has been, a smoker, in which case a yearly chest X-ray is a must. If the woman has been a heavy smoker, then it is possible that twice-yearly chest X-rays may be indicated.

For the menopausal woman who has just begun a strenuous sport such as jogging, stress testing is indicated just as it is with her male counterpart. In addition, every physical examination should include a breast examination. Women already should be conducting self-examination of the breasts at least once a month, but the yearly physical examination needs to include a check on her findings by the physician.

8

You and Your Fitness Program

There are two hurdles to overcome in order to get physically fit. First is keeping up the desire to become fit, and second is finding the time to achieve and maintain fitness. The desire to become fit has to come from within you. We can only tell you what to expect from being fit. Finding the time for an exercise program also can be difficult, but don't forget that it is important to have an activity period at least three times a week. Here are several suggestions for various circumstances.

Fitting Activity into Active Days

If you are a housewife with children in school, you probably can find a time during the day to carry on your activity program. Your hours tend to be more flexible, so you can get involved in programs at the community recreation centers, in the YWCA, schools, colleges, or universities. If you have young children at home, here are some suggestions for finding time to exercise.

1. Work out a schedule with your husband so that three days a week for an hour each he stays with the children while you participate in your activity. This could either be early in the morning before breakfast or in the evening when he is home from work.

2. Hire a babysitter for one hour, three days a week, if you can afford it.

3. Take turns with your neighbors watching each other's

children for an hour each. If several mothers with young children live in the neighborhood and a few of you like to do the same activity, pair up with each other while the other parents watch your children, and then switch.

4. Run through a basic exercise program when the children are napping, or get the older ones to do it with you.

5. Do some basic exercises during the week and on the weekends bicycle with your family, play tennis with your husband or friends, or participate in whatever your favorite activity is.

A word of caution is necessary. If you have small children, try not to take them with you when you are participating in an activity that they can't do or that prohibits keeping them busy. You will spend most of the time watching, chasing, or worrying about them instead of concentrating on yourself and your activity. If this is the *only* choice open to you, then you will have to do the best you can, but it is a less than ideal situation, and we urge you to try to find another alternative.

If you are a woman working in industry and have access to fitness centers provided by the company, by all means use them. Fortunately, more and more industries are building gyms, jogging paths, and tennis and racquetball courts for their employees' use. They have found that they get better production from their employees if the employees have a period of physical activity during the working day. Unfortunately, some industries allow only their executives into the recreation areas. This is sad but, hopefully, changing. If you are in this situation, try to persuade your superiors to allow you and your coworkers to be able to use the recreational facilities too.

If you do have access to a recreational facility at your place of work, put aside a part of your day for your fitness program. The lunch hour is a good time to be active, and you might find that after a period of physical activity you aren't as hungry as you usually are after just sitting for hours. You are also able to function more efficiently for the rest of the day.

Employees of colleges and universities, where recreational facilities are usually in abundance, can set aside a certain time each day for physical activity, either before work, during the lunch hour, or after work. This job location is usually excellent, because many times there will be some kind of exercise program going on through the physical education or recreation department.

Those of you who work eight to five or nine to six daily will have to find a time in that schedule to carry out your activity program. You·could get up very early, exercise, shower, and go to work. In the evenings you have more hours, so you could be active directly after work or later on in the evening.

For the most part, people seem to prefer exercise before dinner and, of course, this is better for you. Then again, if you play on a volleyball team or bowling team, you have to participate at whatever times have been scheduled. Sometimes this is late enough for you to eat and rest before engaging in vigorous activity.

If you are working for a small firm with no facilities, check out what facilities are nearby, such as schools, recreation centers, or fitness centers. Persuade your boss to let you accrue your coffee break time and take an hour and a half for lunch. If none of these work, you will just have to fit your activity program in before or after work.

There are very few *good* excuses for not participating in an activity or exercise program. One common bad excuse is "I'm too tired when I get home." Most of the time this is from mental fatigue or boredom, and not from physical fatigue. If you have been sitting all day the best thing for you would be to get up and get your body moving, your heart pumping, and your blood circulating. You will be surprised how much better you will feel.

At least give it a try and see if we are right. It's just having the discipline to get started that is hard. As soon as you come home, change into your activity clothes and begin your activity *immediately,* even if this is the last thing you want to do. Most of the time you will feel 100 percent better afterward.

If you work on your feet all day, find an activity you can do off your feet. Some examples are basic exercises, bicycling, weight training, swimming, or other water sports (except water skiing).

Another bad excuse is "I go to work too early." Our response is, what about the late afternoon or evening hours? Recreational centers, YWCAs, fitness centers, and the like are open all day and evening and there is always something going on.

A further excuse is "I work odd shifts." Even if you work unusual hours, try to set aside about one hour three days a week to be active. If you never quite know when you'll be working, try to get into a routine of exercising when you get up or as soon as you go home, regardless of what time it is. By the way, it is best not to engage in strenuous activity and then go right to bed because you need time to relax. If you must do it this way, however, a warm shower or bath would help relax you before you go to bed.

The excuse "I'm too old to be active" is the poorest excuse of all. No one is ever too old to be active. In fact, if you look at older people, the ones who are active look younger than they really are. If you feel good and your periodic medical checkups are good, there is no reason why you cannot participate in some activity *as long as you begin gradually and sensibly.*

Women who live in the city have a much easier time finding an organized activity than women who live in less populous communities. There are more activities to choose from and more facilities available. Women who live elsewhere will have to make the most of what they have in their area, whether it be bowling alleys, skating rinks, schools, community centers, or the like.

The winter is a harder time to get your activity program under way than is the summer. With the long, warm summer evenings, it is easier to want to get outside and be active. Once again, you will have to discipline yourself to keep it up whatever the season. Most active women agree that it takes about six months of hard self-discipline to get into an activity routine. Then it becomes so much a part of your life that you miss it if you aren't active.

Family Fitness

If you are a working woman with a family and are concerned that you don't spend enough time with them, there are several activities you can do to achieve fitness and be with your family at the same time. The kinds of activities you can do with your family depend upon the age of your children.

Bicycling is a good family activity, either with the kids cycling with you or, if they are small, riding in a children's bicycle seat behind you. Jogging is a good group activity if the children are old enough to keep up (unless you go to a track where they can go at their own pace and you can still watch them). If you have a large family, volleyball is an excellent game, and involve the neighborhood, too, with certain days set aside for practice or games. Badminton is a vigorous game (if played correctly) requiring a smaller area than volleyball and fewer players. Tennis can be a good family activity if the children are old enough to play a decent game with you. Most water sports, also, can be family activities.

Engaging in family activities promotes togetherness and shows your children that physical activity should be an important part of their daily lives. The earlier they learn this, the earlier they can begin to find their own activities to enjoy and pursue to a high level of skill.

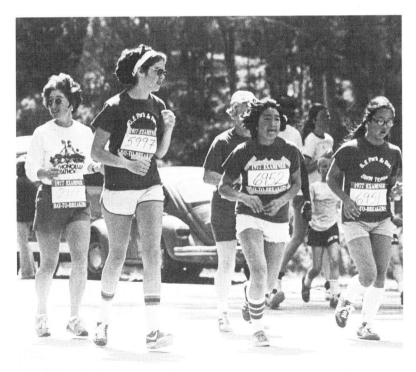

Running

Examples of Activity Programs

Occasionally you read how working women keep their figures and stay in good physical condition. These women spend their lunch hours in ballet classes or fitness centers or do something physically active and then eat a very light lunch afterward. It can be done! Here are some examples of how several women have established activity programs. Hopefully one of these ideas will inspire you and help you find a way to begin your program. you find a way to begin your program.

Joan

Joan is a housewife and mother of two school-age girls, who also works an eight-hour day five days a week. She is an avid bicycle racer and tourist. When she is in training for races, she is up at 5:30 a.m., riding the stationary rollers (moving cylinders on which a bike can be balanced to allow indoor riding) for an hour. Then she rides her bike to work and home again at the end of the day. After work, if she doesn't ride the rollers again, she rides twenty to twenty-five miles. She rides about 200 miles a week. (Her husband is a bicyclist, too, and they take turns racing, touring, and taking care of the children.)

Mandy

A mother of three very young children, Mandy's activity time is greatly limited. She and her husband have worked out a schedule so that she can go to the nearby university three times a week for the 6:30 a.m. exercise class. Two other evenings each week she attends an hour-long ballet class offered by the community recreation center. These hours are perfect for them because it is compatible with her husband's schedule so they do not have to hire a babysitter.

Maureen

Maureen is a computer systems manager who has a difficult time finding an hour to exercise. When she can get away from her office at noon, she swims laps for thirty minutes. If she

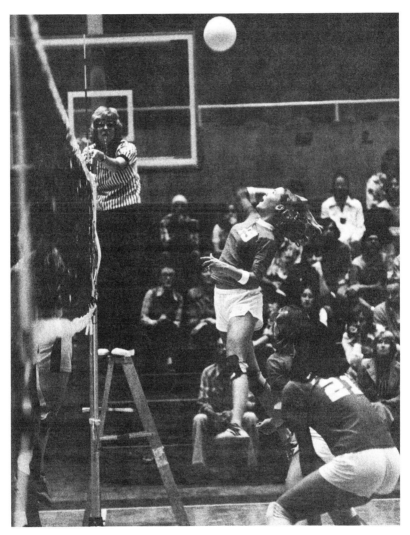

Volleyball

doesn't swim during the day, she jogs after work. On weekends she tries to jog or ride her bicycle.

Sally

A principal of a large high school, Sally joined a fitness center which she tries to attend two or three times a week. She says the only way she will get some activity is by paying money for it.

Betsy

Betsy is the mother of a small child and is employed as a part-time librarian. She makes her jogging time coincide with the time her husband can be at home. She runs about three miles regularly, and on weekends enters local races, cheered on by her husband and son.

Judy

Judy is an assistant to a dean in a large university. She saves up her coffee breaks and takes an extra long lunch hour to jog about four miles. Luckily, her boss is also a runner who runs during the lunch hour, so there are no problems if she happens to be late or if she wants to start earlier than usual.

Dorothy

Dorothy, a mother and grandmother, is a jogger. She is also head of the counseling service at a large university. Her lunch hours are reserved for jogging two miles and she gardens on the weekends.

Karen

A math professor and mother of a small boy, Karen stays active in all kinds of sports, especially swimming, golf, and tennis. She plays in tennis leagues in the summer and fall, and during the winter as often as possible.

And, last but not least, the two authors:

Gail

Gail is lucky in that teaching in the physical education department at a university allows her access to all kinds of facilities. Generally, she runs or swims during the lunch hour, and on weekends she takes bicycle tours.

Chris

Chris, a general surgeon and teacher in a medical school, has difficulty finding time to exercise. She plays tennis whenever she can, and during the summer months she plays softball, her favorite activity.

After reading about these women, you might wonder if they all have perfect figures. The answer is *no!* The point, however, is that these women realize that some type of physical activity is important to their well-being and thus have made it an important part of their lives. Granted, some of these women are more active than others, but they all know how much better it makes them feel when they are physically active.

Obtaining Results

Many women become upset when they don't see results right away or even after several weeks of being in some type of an activity program. Several reasons can be cited for this lack of results. First, if you are just doing a basic exercise program, noticeable results will take much longer than if you are in some type of vigorous activity. Another reason is that you may not have participated as vigorously as you should have for the proper length of time. Thirdly, you may not have cut down on your eating as you should have.

Don't think that just because you were active for an hour permits you to have a chocolate sundae "since it will even out anyway." Not true! You are eating many more calories than you burned. It takes *at least six weeks* for any noticeable results to occur *assuming you have exercised regularly and have cut back on your food intake.* Remember that muscle weighs more than fat, and as you are replacing the fat with muscle, your weight will not change until you burn off that excess fat. It takes a long time. You will notice a loss of inches sooner than a loss of weight.

Be honest with yourself and your exercise program as you try to lose weight and become fit. Answer the following questions as honestly as you can. If you can answer "yes" to all the questions, you will get the results you desire.

1. Do you exercise at least three times a week?
2. Do you exercise for at least thirty minutes at each exercise session?

3. Do you exercise at 70 percent of your maximum heart rate for at least thirty minutes?
4. Do you exercise with as much vigor as possible?
5. Do you exercise toward all three components of fitness (muscular strength and endurance, flexibility, and cardiovascular endurance)?
6. Do you reduce your food intake?

We hope the information presented in this book will set you straight about your body and why some type of physical activity should be a part of your life. We encourage you to find some activity you like and to participate in it as actively as possible within your time schedule.

Take a positive attitude, making your activity program something you *want* to do and not something you *have* to do. Once you become fit, maintain it. It's much easier to stay in shape than to get in shape, so don't lose what you worked so hard for. We promise you that although it may not be fun all the time, it will be much of the time, and your whole being will be enhanced.

Good luck!!!

Appendix

Charts

Women's Caloric Expenditure During Exercise
Daily Fitness Progress Chart
Daily Food Intake
Muscular Strength and Endurance
Flexibility
Cardiovascular Tests
Body Composition
Estimate Your Overall Fitness
Measurement Chart
Desirable Weights for Heights
Calorie Allowances for Individuals

Women's Caloric Expenditure During Exercise
(in calories per minute)

Bicycling*
5.5 m.p.h.	2.1
9.4 m.p.h.	6.0
13.1 m.p.h.	9.5

Running
12-min. mile (5 m.p.h.)	8.4
8-min. mile (7.5 m.p.h.)	12.4
6-min. mile (10 m.p.h.)	16.1
5-min. mile (12 m.p.h.)	20.0

Swimming
25 yds./min.	5.1
50 yds./min.*	10.4

Hiking
Level road (3½ m.p.h.)	5.6
Downhill (2½ m.p.h.)	3.5
Uphill, 5% (3½ m.p.h.)	6.5
Uphill, 15% (3½ m.p.h.)	12.5

*On level roads. Add 20-50% for grades up to 5%.

(Sources: *Food: The Yearbook of Agriculture*, 1959, USDA; R. Passmore and J.V.G.A. Durnin, *Physiological Review*, 35 (1955): 801; Jean Mayer, *Overweight* (Englewood Cliffs, N.J.: Prentice-Hall, 1968); and Brian J. Sharkey, *Fitness and Work Capacity*, Forest Service 315, USDA, 1977.)

DAILY FITNESS PROGRESS CHART

	PRESENT WEIGHT	ACTIVITY	DURATION OF ACTIVITY	CAL. BURNED (Est. from Chart)	CAL. CONSUMED (Estimate)	DESIRED WEIGHT
Monday						
Tuesday						
Wednesday						
Thursday						
Friday						
Saturday						
Sunday						
Comments:						
Monday						
Tuesday						
Wednesday						
Thursday						
Friday						
Saturday						
Sunday						
Comments:						

DAILY FOOD INTAKE

	MONDAY	TUESDAY	WEDNESDAY	THURSDAY	FRIDAY	SATURDAY	SUNDAY
BREAKFAST							
LUNCH							
DINNER							
SNACKS							

MUSCULAR STRENGTH AND ENDURANCE

	STRENGTH P/F	ENDURANCE No. of Repetitions
1. Sit-Ups	_____	_____
2. Push-Ups	_____	_____
3. Chins	_____	_____
4. Back Arch	_____	_____
5. 1/2 Knee Bend	_____	_____
No. Passed	_____	
No. Failed	_____	
Score		
	(5=Ex; 4=G; 3=F; 2-1=P)	
Areas to Work On	_____	

FLEXIBILITY

TEST	P/F
1. Toe Touch	_____
2. Knee-Head Touch	_____
3. Hand Clasp	_____
4. Toe-Heel Touch	_____
5. Calf Stretch	_____
6. Heel-Seat Touch	_____
7. Side Bend	_____
8. Rocker	_____
No. Passed	_____
No. Failed	_____
Score	
	(7-8=Ex; 5-6=G; 3-4=F; 1-2=P)
Areas to Work On	_____

CARDIOVASCULAR TESTS

SCORE

Revised Katch Step Test _____

*Swimming _____

*Walking/Running _____

*Bicycling _____

*Rope Skipping _____

(*From Cooper's *The New Aerobics*)

BODY COMPOSITION

P/F

Skin Thickness Behind Upper Arm

   1 inch — F _____

   1 inch — P _____

ESTIMATE YOUR OVERALL FITNESS

	EXCEL	GOOD	FAIR	POOR
Muscle Strength and Endurance	_____	_____	_____	_____
Flexibility	_____	_____	_____	_____
Cardiovascular Endurance	_____	_____	_____	_____
Body Composition		_____		_____
TOTAL FITNESS ESTIMATE	_____	_____	_____	_____

MEASUREMENT CHART

1 – Calf
2 – Thigh
3 – Hips
4 – Waist
5 – Chest
6 – Upper Arm

Take measurements with tape measurement every two weeks. Measure at heaviest part of each area.

DATE											
1											
2											
3											
4											
5											
6											

DESIRABLE WEIGHTS FOR HEIGHTS

Height (in inches)	Weight (in pounds)	
	Men	Women
58	---	112 + 11
60	125 + 13	116 + 12
62	130 + 13	121 + 12
64	135 + 14	128 + 13
66	142 + 14	135 + 14
68	150 + 15	142 + 14
70	158 + 15	150 + 15
72	167 + 17	150 + 16
74	178 + 18	----

CALORIE ALLOWANCES FOR INDIVIDUALS

Desirable Weight

Calorie Allowance

Men

Pounds	25 years	45 years	65 years
110	2500	2350	1950
121	2700	2550	2150
132	2850	2700	2250
143	3000	2800	2350
154	3200	3000	2550
165	3400	3200	2700
176	3550	3350	2800
187	3700	3500	2900

Women

Pounds	25 years	45 years	65 years
88	1750	1650	1400
99	1900	1800	1500
110	2050	1950	1600
121	2200	2050	1750
128	2300	2200	1800
132	2350	2200	1850
143	2500	2350	2000
154	2600	2450	2050
165	2750	2600	2150

Recommended Reading

Beinhorn, George. *Food for Fitness*. Mountain View: World Publications, 1975.

Couch, Jean. *Runner's World Yoga Book*. Mountain View: World Publications, 1979.

Darden, Ellington. *Especially for Women*. West Point, New York: Leisure Press, 1977.

Editors of *Runner's World* Magazine. *The Complete Diet Guide*. Mountain View: World Publication, 1978.

Editors of *Runner's World* Magazine. *The Complete Woman Runner*. Mountain View: World Publications, 1978.

Getchell, Bud. *Physical Fitness: A Way of Life*. New York: John Wiley & Sons, Inc., 1976.

Henderson, Joe. *Jog, Run, Race*. Mountain View: World Publications, 1977.

Henderson, Joe. *Run Farther, Run Faster*. Mountain View: World Publications, 1979.

Higdon, Hal. *Beginner's Running Guide*. Mountain View: World Publications, 1978.

Hockey, Robert. *Physical Fitness: The Pathway to Healthful Living*. St. Louis: The C. V. Mosby Co., 1977.

Jensen, Clayne, and Fisher, A. Garth. *Scientific Basis of Athletic Conditioning*. Philadelphia: Lea and Febiger, 1975.

Johnson, P. B., Updyke, W. F., Schaefer, M., and Stolberg, D. C. *Sport, Exercise, and You*. New York: Holt, Rinehart and Winston, 1975.

Katch, F. I., and McArdle, W. D. *Nutrition, Weight Control, and Exercise*. Boston: Houghton Mifflin Co., 1977.

Klafs, Carl, and Lyon, Joan. *The Female Athlete*. St. Louis: The C. V. Mosby Co., 1978.

Kramer, Jack. *Beginner's Racquetball*. Mountain View: World Publications, 1979.

MacIntyre, Christine. *Complete Women's Weight Training Guide*. Mountain View: World Publications, 1979.

Mirkin, Gabe, and Hoffman, Marshall. *The Sportsmedicine Book*. Boston: Little, Brown and Company, 1978.

Novich, Max M., and Taylor, Buddy. *Training and Conditioning of Athletes*. Philadelphia: Lea & Febiger, 1972.

Reynolds, Bill. *Complete Weight Training Book*. Mountain View: World Publications, 1976.

Sheehan, George. *Medical Advice for Runners*. Mountain View: World Publications, 1978.

Sheehan, George. *Doctor Sheehan on Running*. Mountain View: World Publications, 1975.

Smith, Nathan. *Food for Sport*. Palo Alto: Bull Publishing Co., 1976.

Thomas, Vaughan. *Science and Sport*. Boston: Little, Brown and Co., 1970.

Ullyot, Joan. *Women's Running*. Mountain View: World Publications, 1976.

Uram, Paul. *The Complete Stretching Book*. Mountain View: World Publications, 1979.

Wilmore, Jack. *Athletic Training and Physical Fitness*. Boston: Allyn and Bacon, Inc., 1977.

About The Authors

Gail Shierman, Ph.D.

Dr. Shierman attended Russell Sage College and the University of Massachusetts and received her Ph.D. from Texas Woman's University. She has taught physical education at the junior high school, high school, and college levels, and presently is an assistant professor of health, physical education, and recreation at the University of Oklahoma. Published in several sports and health magazines, her teaching and research interests are in the area of biomechanics and kinesiology. She swims or runs daily and bicycle-tours on weekends.

Christine Haycock, M.D.

Dr. Haycock received her M.D. degree from State University of New York, Downstate Medical Center, and had postgraduate training at Walter Reed Army Medical Center and Brooke Army Hospital. She also is a graduate of the Army Command and General Staff College and the United States Army War College. Presently an associate professor of surgery at the New Jersey College of Medicine and Dentistry, a fellow of the American College of Sports Medicine, and a member of the editorial board of *The Physician and Sportsmedicine* magazine, Haycock is a multipublished author and frequent lecturer on the subjects of trauma and women as athletes.